ADA: TOWARDS MATU

CW01072413

Studies in
Computer and Communications Systems

Volume 6

Editors
Arvind (MIT)
Ulrich Herzog (Universität Erlangen)
Richard Muntz (UCLA)
Brigitte Plateau (IMAG, Grenoble)
Ken Sevcik (University of Toronto)
Satish Tripathi (University of Maryland)

ISSN: 0927-5444

Ada: Towards Maturity

edited by

L. Collingbourne

IOS Press
1993
Amsterdam • Oxford • Washington, DC • Tokyo

ISBN 90 5199 142 8
ISSN 0927-5444
Library of Congress Catalog Card Number: 93-061134

Publisher:

IOS Press
Van Diemenstraat 94
1013 CN Amsterdam
Netherlands

Sole distributor in the UK and Ireland:

IOS Press/Lavis Marketing
73 Lime Walk
Headington
Oxford OX3 7AD
England

Distributor in the USA and Canada:

IOS Press, Inc.
P.O. Box 10558
Burke, VA 22009-0558
USA

Distributor in Japan:

Kaigai Publications, Ltd.
21 Kanda Tsukasa-Cho 2-Chome
Chiyoda-Ku
Tokyo 101
Japan

Printed in the Netherlands

Preface

Ada is moving towards maturity. It is no longer the new language that controversially challenged programming concepts and fuelled philosophical debate; Ada is well understood, widely used and has proven benefits in thousands of applications. Compilers and tools have been developed to support its use on a wide range of platforms. They have the performance, reliability and CASE support to match other popular languages such as C and C++. Ada is therefore becoming the programming language of choice in an ever growing range of applications from information systems to real-time systems. As a reflection of Ada's maturing status, the focus of technical debate has shifted from discussion of language-specific issues, towards a more outward looking concern to meet the practical requirements of real applications. The major features of the Ada 9X language revision process address this outward focus. Object Oriented Programming (OOP), more maintainable program libraries, more flexible real-time facilities, and consideration of distributed and safety critical systems, all respond to specific requirements. Feedback from experience of using "Ada 83" provides practical testimony to the benefits of language and also provides important input into the language's revision. But perhaps the most exciting and challenging area for Ada is that it is probably the best high level programming language for use in safety critical computer systems. As these systems become more complex and are integrated with other management systems, Ada supports the good software engineering practice and improved productivity that are critical to their implementation.

Both the Ada UK International Conference and this book focus on these three themes of Ada's maturing status: Ada 9X revision, application to high integrity systems and feedback from practical applications.

This book is of interest to both current and intending practitioners of Ada.

Lawrence Collingbourne

Contents

Editorial

Lawrence Collingbourne

EDS-Scicon, Pembroke Broadway, Camberley, Surrey GU15 3XD

1. Introduction

This year is the tenth anniversary of the current standard of the Ada programming language, ANSI/MIL-STD-1815A. It is also the year when the draft text of its first major revision will be published. Ada is moving towards maturity. No longer the new language that controversially challenged programming concepts and fuelled philosophical debate; Ada is well understood, widely used and has proven benefits in thousands of applications. Compilers and tools have been developed to support its use on a wide range of platforms. They have the performance, reliability and CASE support to match other popular languages such as C and C++. Ada is therefore becoming the programming language of choice in an ever growing range of applications from information systems to real-time systems.

As a reflection of Ada's maturing status, the focus of technical debate has shifted from discussion of language-specific issues, towards a more outward looking concern to meet the practical requirements of real applications. The major features of the Ada 9X language revision process address this outward focus. Object Oriented Programming (OOP), more maintainable program libraries, more flexible real-time facilities, and consideration of distributed and safety critical systems, all respond to specific requirements. The revision process began with a requirements capture phase and has continued at each stage to relate proposed changes to the agreed requirements. Feedback from experience of using "Ada 83" provides practical testimony to the benefits of language and also provides important input into the language's revision. But perhaps the most exciting and challenging area for Ada is that it is probably the best high level programming language for use in safety critical computer systems. As these systems become more complex and are integrated with other management systems, Ada supports the good software engineering practice and improved productivity that are critical to their implementation.

Both the Ada UK International Conference and this book focus on these three themes of Ada's maturing status: Ada 9X revision, application to high integrity systems and feedback from practical applications.

2. Ada 9X Revision

The Ada 9X revision is a mammoth task. Without taking into account any new requirements, there are hundreds of questions of interpretation and suggested revisions to consider. Ada needs to be easier to use and some of its complexities and inconsistencies need rationalisation, and there are pressing requirements for new capabilities to meet specific requirements. The revisions interact with each other and existing language implementations in complex ways, making it difficult to bring everything together in an accurate and unambiguous language definition.

Ada 9X is therefore both an opportunity and a threat to the maturity of Ada. Failure to meet the new requirements would leave Ada poorly equipped to meet the needs of the 90s. Excessive change would de-stabilise the maturity of the language: it would be difficult to apply the new features and implementations might regress in reliability, performance or time to market. Ada 9X must be accomplished quickly, efficiently and effectively if the revision process is to be a success.

All this comes to a head as the language definition is published and debated. In the meantime it is important that attention is kept firmly on the revisions which will enhance Ada's application and maturity as a programming language. The Ada UK International Conference papers in this book address some of these important issues.

Ada is well established as a real-time programming language in the defence arena, but until recently has not been seen as a natural language to use for development of "open systems". The UNIX family of operating systems has recently been extended to include real-time facilities and to support distributed, multiprocessing systems. Karen Sielski shows in her paper how Ada run-time facilities have been implemented to make Ada in established part of this open environment.

One of the problems besetting software engineering is the continual re-invention of design solutions to well-known problems. This increases both development and maintenance costs and reduces reliability. In mature engineering industries, such as car manufacturing, products are largely constructed from a set of individual components, most of which are re-used across the product range and even across the industry. Anthony Gargaro shows how Ada 9X facilities for object oriented programming and distribution could enable a quantum leap in maturity to component-based software engineering.

In the last two papers on the Ada 9X theme, Bill Taylor reviews the proposed language revision against the agreed requirements as a check on progress to date, and John English provides a comparative review of the object oriented programming features with those of C++ to provide some practical lessons on how to use the new features successfully.

3. Application to High Integrity Systems

Computers are being increasingly used to enhance the effectiveness of more and more systems upon which our safety and welfare depend, such as vehicles, signalling, power generation and security. When computers were first introduced into these high integrity systems their operation was kept simple. The amount of software upon which the safe operation of the system depended was kept very small and it was uncommon for a high level language to be used in its development. However, as the benefits of using computers have been demonstrated and confidence in their operation has been established, their functionality is growing very rapidly. For example, on military aircraft the size of computer programs has typically grown an order of magnitude in one generation, so that aircraft currently in development in Europe and the USA will have megabytes of code controlling almost all on-board systems. Both civil and military aircraft are now "fly-by-computer".

It is now no longer sufficient for the software for these high integrity systems to be developed by "hand-crafted" techniques in a low-level language or machine code. Not only has the amount of safety-critical code increased, much more significantly it is becoming inter-operable with less critical systems management functions. High integrity computer systems are in fact multilevel critical in a complex manner, requiring a integrated development methodology from requirements definition and analysis right through to the executable program code.

Ada is probably the best high level language to use in high integrity systems. It was created to satisfy the software engineering requirements and real-time nature of such systems, and has the necessary tool support required to for the software engineering life cycle. However, compared to other widely available (and therefore well-tried and trusted) languages, it is the most stable, well-defined and rigorously validated language available.

The second major theme of the Ada UK International Conference and this book is the application of Ada to the programming of such systems. John McDermid introduces the subject with an excellent overview of the principles and problems of programming safety critical systems in Ada, identifying the key properties that must be satisfied to meet defence requirements. The most important technique identified in the defence community is formal design methods that use rational and mathematical proofs to establish the absence of errors. In order for these to be successfully applied, it is imperative to provide tools to help automate much of the process and thereby increase productivity. Further papers in the book take up specific problems associated with establishing adequate levels of confidence in Ada programs economically.

One of the major contributions Ada has made to programming has been to recognise that errors do occur at run-time and therefore to provide a way of handling these by means of exceptions. However, run-time errors are generally fatal to the correct operation of real-time control systems. Jon Garnsworthy takes up the issue of proving that such run-time errors will not occur in a high integrity program and describes how tools could be used to automate much of the verification required.

Two papers review advances in formal design methods for Ada and provide further contribution to the unresolved debate on how tools might be used to simplify the formal development process and make it more efficient. Michael Hinchey introduces a formal method that can be applied to real-time Ada systems, addressing the complex issue of proving the correctness of multithreaded programs. Paul Taylor takes up the theme of how tools may be used to support the analysis required to verify the refinement process in the development life cycle.

Finally, Roderick Chapman takes up the corollary of the second paper, namely to allow run-time errors to be handled safely in real-time systems. He proposes an analysis method that might relax what has been a significant constraint and area of risk in high integrity systems. In particular, this could allow Ada exceptions to be used to provide finer grained recovery procedures than can otherwise be supported.

4. Feedback from Practical Applications

Something that is mature is well thought out and fully developed, and so there is no better test for the maturity of a programming language than to receive feedback on its practical use and application. Over the last ten years it has to be said that the feedback from Ada applications has been mixed, but improving. The implementations of Ada have taken a few years to mature, but now have the performance and reliability of other languages. Ada has also introduced new concepts and capabilities that need experience to use effectively, and which shift the balance of development effort to earlier in the life cycle. There is now a wealth of such experience available through international conferences such as Ada UK's. Although originally seen as a real-time programming language, programmers were slow to take up Ada's tasking features for both the reasons above, but also because of lack of theoretical support for the predictability of asynchronous scheduling mechanisms. This is now well understood and Ada 9X is taking abstract real-time support in the language a step further with protected records.

Four papers in the Ada UK International Conference and this book provide feedback from practical application of Ada to real systems. Caroline Langensiepen describes some of the pitfalls that can be encountered when designing large Ada programs and provides some recommendations for avoiding them. Simon Barker describes his experience of designing and developing a systems trials facility which features an OSF/Motif Graphical User Interface (GUI) developed in Ada. John Smart has found a gap in the Ada predefined library in the area of text formatting and describes the implementation of a package to provide the missing functionality.

Finally Chris Hall presents the paper that best demonstrates Ada's growth to maturity of all the papers in this book. Faced with the need to develop a simple application on a cheap personal computer that required the latest graphics user interfaces, he chose Ada. The application tugs the heart strings of every parent: the real-time monitoring of babies as part of research into sudden infant death syndrome. Ada has delivered performance, reliability, capability and perhaps the most intangible of all: hope for the future.

Ada: Towards Maturity
Ed. L. Collingbourne
IOS Press 1993

Implementing Ada 83 and Ada 9X Using Solaris Threads

Karen L. Sielski

SunPro, 2525 Garcia Ave. UMTV 12-40 Mountain View, CA. 94043

Abstract

This paper describes several implementations of Ada runtime systems on the Solaris architecture, with emphasis on the use of Solaris Threads. It begins by discussing "traditional" Ada 83 implementations with an Ada specific runtime. The Solaris multithread architecture and the implementation of SPARCompiler Ada using Solaris Threads are then described. Finally, key Ada 9X features are described, and the feasibility of implementing these new features using Solaris Threads is discussed.

1. Overview

The Ada language was introduced in the early 1980's to reduce software development and maintenance costs, improve software reusability, and provide a standard language to support real-time and multiprocessing system development. In the 10 years that have elapsed since Ada was adopted there have been many advances in software engineering practices. In addition, years of practical experience with the Ada language have exposed areas of the standard which can be improved. In order to take advantage of the knowledge acquired since its introduction, the language is being revised. Ada 9X is the designation for the revision of the Ada 83 language. Major changes in Ada 9X include inheritance to improve object-oriented programming in Ada, hierarchical Ada libraries to enhance support for programming in the large, and asynchronous communication for improved real-time capabilities.

The Ada 9X process has been progressing for several years, and produced a requirements document in December of 1990. This document is currently being translated into specific language rules by the Ada 9X Mapping/Revision Team. The Ada 9X revision will be composed of a "core" language specification, a library specification, and the specificiation of optional annexes. The annexes include: systems programming, real-time systems, distributed systems, information systems, safety and security systems, and numerical systems.

This paper describes the Ada 83 tasking model, the Solaris 2 multithread architecture, experiences with SPARCompiler Ada using Solaris threads to implement the Ada 83 tasking model, and changes to the tasking model in Ada 9X, with emphasis on implementation using Solaris threads. It's focus is primarily on changes to the core language specification, with coverage of some portions of the systems programming annex and real-time annex. The systems programming annex supports low-level features such as machine code, interrupt handling, task identification, and shared variables. The real-time annex has the systems programming annex as a pre-requisite and contains specifications for task priorities and scheduling, entry queue policies, dynamic priorities, preemptive abort, and time and delays.

2. Ada 83

The Ada tasking mechanism is a key aspect of the language and provides the construct for achieving parallel execution, communication, and synchronization. Ada tasks can be viewed as independent, concurrent operations that communicate with each other by passing messages. Ada tasking provides the high-level, standard interface to underlying operating system mechanisms used to implement parallel task execution. Tasks are designed to execute simultaneously in a multiprocessor system or with interleaved execution on a uniprocessor.

The Ada tasking model has been criticized as being inadequate for many applications, especially those which have time-critical requirements. The criticisms fall into two categories, those which originate from the limitations and deficiencies in the definition of the Ada tasking model itself, and those which are based on the inefficient implementations that exist. In many time-critical applications, deficient Ada tasking has caused users to abandon the tasking model in favor of implementation-specific mechanisms, thus losing many of Ada's portability benefits.

3. Ada 83 Implementations

Many early implementations of Ada on UNIX were inadequate for time-critical systems due to the real-time deficiencies of the underlying operating systems. The best approach in implementing an Ada runtime is to map Ada tasks to entities schedulable by the operating system and let the operating system handle task scheduling, synchronization and communication. To implement Ada task priority specifications requires an operating system which supports static process priorities while allowing the user to manipulate process priorities if necessary. And in order to implement an efficient tasking rendezvous mechanism, it is almost essential to use shared memory to minimize overhead and provide acceptable performance.

Given the portability issues, high overhead, and functional difficulties in scheduling Ada tasks as UNIX processes, most vendors choose the alternative approach, which is to assign a single UNIX process to the entire Ada program and have the Ada runtime handle task scheduling and communication. Context switch overhead is minimal in this approach because the UNIX kernel is not involved. The major problem with this method is that whenever the single UNIX process is preempted, all of the tasks in the Ada program are also preempted because they are part of the same UNIX process.

USER PROCESS

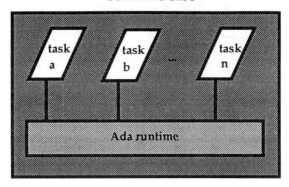

Figure 1."Traditional" Ada Process

4.   Solaris 2 Multithreading and Multiprocessing

One of the major new features of Solaris 2, based on UNIX SVR4 from UNIX International, is support for time-critical applications.   SVR4 contains time-critical features such as fixed priority real-time processes, user process priority manipulation, and high resolution timers. In addition to these standard UNIX SVR4 real-time features, Solaris 2 has many value-added features, the most important of which is a multithreaded environment.

To achieve a completely preemptive kernel and deterministic dispatch latency, the system has been re-architected with multithreading and multiprocessing as a main goal. A key aspect of the multithreaded approach is that it allows the system to run efficiently on uniprocessor as well as multiprocessor systems.   Solaris 2 is a symmetric multiprocessing system with significant performance advantages over asymmetric models, especially as the number of processors increases.

5.   Threads

A thread is a flow of control within a single UNIX process address space. Solaris threads provide a light-weight form of concurrent task, allowing multiple threads of control in a common address space, with minimal scheduling and communication overhead. Threads share the same address space, file descriptors, data structures, and operating system state. A thread has a program counter and a stack to keep track of local variables and return addresses. Threads interact through the use of global variables and thread synchronization operations.

Threads execute independently and are the lightest entity schedulable by the kernel. A thread can be scheduled by the kernel via a lightweight process, but the kernel does not "know" about them. Threads can be preempted at any time by other threads.   Threads can be created, destroyed, blocked, etc. without involving the kernel, providing very fast thread-to-thread context switch times. Threads are executed by lightweight processes, which are known to the kernel. A thread can execute a kernel call at any time.

6.　Lightweight Processes (LWPs)

Like threads, LWPs share an address space, but unlike threads, LWPs are known to the kernel. A context switch between LWPs involves the kernel but does not require an address state switch. The overhead is less than a UNIX process context switch, but more than a thread context switch.

When a thread executes a kernel call, it remains bound to the same LWP for the duration of the system call. If the kernel call blocks, the thread and its lightweight process blocks. Other LWPs may execute other threads in the program, including the execution of kernel calls. In a multiprocessor system, LWPs can be scheduled to run on separate processors but all threads associated with that LWP must run on the same processor as the LWP.

One LWP is created by the kernel when a program is started, and it starts executing the thread compiled as the main program. Additional threads are created by calls to the thread library. During the execution life of a thread, the thread may permanently bind itself to a single LWP, or it may share its association with any one of several LWPs that constitute a process. An important feature of the Solaris multithreaded architecture is to allow the user to specify how threads should be mapped to LWPs, providing a very high level of flexibility and the ability to meet the requirements of a variety of applications.

For instance, a window controller would best be implemented with multiple threads, one per window, bound to a single LWP. This provides the least amount of overhead when switching from one window to another since the kernel is not involved. On the other hand, a multitasking Ada system with a task dedicated to reading time-critical data from disk is best implemented with a single thread per LWP. In this configuration, only the task blocked on I/O is preempted, and the kernel can schedule other Ada tasks to execute while the I/O task is blocked.

Another example of a system which benefits most from a 1-1 thread-to-LWP mapping is a multiprocessing system in which tasks can be distributed across processors. The single thread-per-LWP configuration allows each task to be assigned to a separate processor.

The programmer is not limited to one scheme or another; all combinations of thread-to-LWP mapping are possible in a single application. Figure 2 depicts most combinations possible within a process. Process 1 is the traditional UNIX process with a single thread attached to a single LWP. Process 2 has multiple threads multiplexed on a single LWP. Process 3 has several threads multiplexed on a lesser number of LWPs. Process 4 has its threads permanently bound to LWPs. Process 5 shows all possibilities: a group of threads multiplexed on a group of LWPs, while having threads bound to LWPs. In addition, one of the LWPs is bound to a CPU.

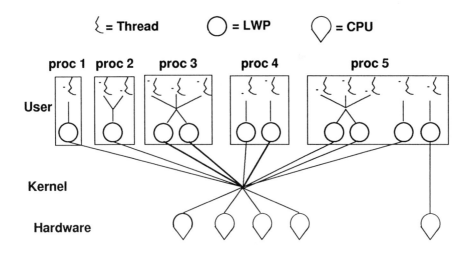

Figure 2.Multithreaded Architecture Examples

7. Synchronization Facilities

Solaris 2 supports different frequencies of interaction and different degrees of concurrency, so provides several synchronization mechanisms with different semantics:

1. mutual exclusion locks
2. counting semaphores
3. condition variables
4. multiple readers, single writer locks

These facilities use synchronization variables in memory. The implementations are very efficient and can synchronize threads within a process as well as between processes. The mutual exclusion lock serializes access to a resource, and is the most efficient mechanism in both memory use and execution time. Condition variables are the next most efficient Solaris threads primitive and allow a program to block on a change of state. The semaphore variable functions on state rather than control so it is easier to use in some circumstances than the condition variable but it uses more memory. The most complex Solaris thread synchronization method is the multiple reader, single writer lock. It is typically used on a resource whose contents are searched more often than they are changed.

8. Signals

Each thread has its own signal mask. Signals are divided into two categories, traps and interrupts. Traps are caused asynchronously by the operation of a thread and are handled only by the thread that caused them. Interrupts are asynchronously generated external to the process. An interrupt is handled by the thread that has it enabled in its signal mask.

9. SPARCompiler Ada and Threads

New versions of SPARCompiler Ada implemented on Solaris 2.2 and higher take full advantage of the new real-time features of Solaris. As have other Ada implementations on Unix, previous versions of SPARCompiler Ada implemented an Ada program as a single UNIX process and performed task scheduling and synchronization in the Ada runtime. With SPARCompiler Ada on Solaris Threads, the Ada runtime implements Ada tasking semantics, and makes calls to the Solaris threads library, which implements operations on threads, mutexes, semaphores, and condition variables. The threads library handles the scheduling of threads for execution on one or more LWPs and facilitates communication between threads. Since all threads execute in a shared UNIX process address space, the tasking implementation is straight forward and overhead is minimal, resulting in very low context switch times. For each Ada task, one Solaris thread is created. The Ada rendezvous mechanism is implemented efficiently using Solaris thread synchronization primitives. If one task blocks, the operating system can schedule another task (thread) to run. The use of Solaris threads also allows SPARCompiler Ada to execute multitasking Ada programs on parallel systems, allocating tasks to processors in an efficient distribution.

The Ada runtime has been completely redesigned to be fast and portable. The redesign allows Ada tasking to be layered on a threads model or to use an Ada-specific microkernel, and provides identical services to the Ada application regardless of the underlying implementation. Figure 3 shows the layers in the new runtime design.

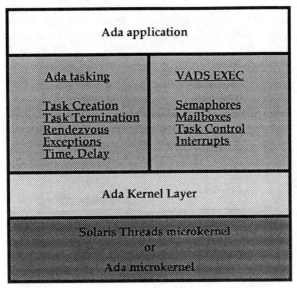

Figure 3. Ada Runtime Layering

At the lowest level is a microkernel, such as Solaris Threads or an Ada specific microkernel. The Ada microkernel implements Ada tasking inside a single UNIX process for architectures which do not have a threads model. On top of the microkernel layer is the Ada kernel layer, which maps microkernel features into the interface required by the Ada tasking and VADS Extensions (VADS_EXEC) layer. In the Solaris Threads environment, the Ada kernel calls the operating system to create and control threads and mutexes, and to interact with the operating-system-defined method of handling traps and interrupts. When the runtime system is ported onto a new microkernel, the main job of porting is writing a new Ada kernel layer for the new microkernel. The Ada tasking and VADS_EXEC layer is common to all implementations of the Ada runtime and provides services directly available to the application program. The Ada tasking layer supports the semantics of the Ada language and the VADS_EXEC layer provides a set of extensions not defined by the Ada language.

In addition to the improved portability of the Ada runtime, the layered design has allowed much of the Ada tasking and semaphore semantics to move to a level higher than the kernel. As a result, many of the common operations are handled without going into the Ada kernel at all and the total throughput of the system is improved.

10. Ada I/O

All Ada I/O packages, *SEQUENTIAL_IO, DIRECT_IO, INTEGER_IO*, and so forth, have been changed to be Ada tasking safe and abort safe. This guarantees atomic file operations on a per task basis and inhibits a task initiating an I/O request from completing by an Ada abort until it finishes.

In the past, *TEXT_IO put* routines could be called from a passive interrupt service routine (ISR) accept body or an ISR handler, because they could not block. Now it is possible to attempt a *put* operation while another task is already doing an I/O operation to the same file and holding its lock. An ISR cannot block waiting for the lock, therefore a *TASKING_ERROR* exception is raised. To allow I/O from an ISR, package *SIMPLE_IO* has been added. This package contains a subset of *TEXT_IO* subprograms and makes unprotected calls to operating system I/O services.

11. Configuration

The Ada runtime creates a thread for each Ada task, but to utilize the full flexibility of the underlying Solaris model, and to provide efficient solutions for real-time applications with a wide range of requirements, controls for the association of threads to LWPs are necessary. Because the optimal mapping may be application specific, the users must be able to configure the system to obtain the most efficient models for their needs. For minimum context switch times (fastest task rendezvous time), a user needs a single LWP, with all tasks (threads) associated with this LWP. In this scenario, context switches are thread-to-thread, with very little overhead. The disadvantage to this model is that a task preempted by the UNIX kernel causes all other tasks associated with this LWP to be preempted. For a system whose requirements cannot tolerate a blocked task preempting other tasks, the user needs a model with an LWP for each task. When a task blocks, the kernel is able to schedule a task associated with a different LWP. And since an LWP is the operating system entity that can be scheduled on distributed processors, maximum use of a multiprocessor system requires at least one LWP per processor.

Several mechanisms in SPARCompiler Ada allow the programmer to configure the association of threads to LWPs. There are three ways to set the level of concurrency in an Ada program:

1. an Ada runtime parameter, CONCURRENCY_LEVEL => x,
2. a runtime system call, *thr_setconcurrency(x)*,
3. and an environment variable, CONCURRENCY_LEVEL.

You can specify whether threads are bound or unbound in two ways:

1. an Ada runtime parameter,

> DEFAULT_TASK_ATTRIBUTES =>
>
>> flags => os_thread.THR_BOUND
>>
>> flags => os_thread.THR_NEW_LWP

2. and a task attribute pragma,

> bound_task_attr : constant ada_krn_defs.task_attr_t :=
>
>> (flags => os_threads.THR_BOUND);
>
> task a is
>
>> pragma task_attributes (bound_task_attr'address);
>
> end;

These configuration methods allow all combinations of thread-to-LWP mapping, and the Solaris thread model allows any number of threads and LWPs in a system; therefore a configuration parameter has no limits. The use of configuration mechanisms by the programmer is optional, and is only reccommended for applications which have specific scheduling requirements.   In general, it is best to use the default configuration and let the threads scheduler optimize the allocation and creation of threads and LWPs. The default configuration does not require any knowledge of the thread model but can still take advantage of the benefits of the system.

Existing standard Ada applications can be compiled and linked with SPARCompiler Ada without being modified; they will take advantage of the underlying thread model, even though it is completely transparent to the end user.

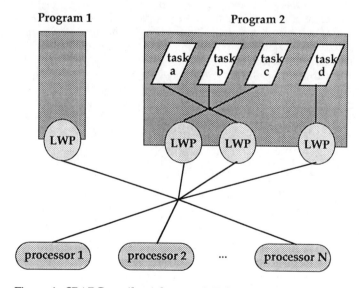

Figure 4. SPARCompiler Ada on an MP System

12. Scheduling

The non-threaded Ada runtime supports an optional scheduling model called time-sliced task scheduling and provides configuration parameters which allow the user to set time- slicing on or off, define the time-slice interval, and specify the maximum task priority to which time-slicing applies.   Time-slice scheduling allows a task of equal priority to preempt an executing task at a specified interval. The time-slice interval is the amount of time a task runs before it can be preempted by the scheduler to see if there are any tasks of equal priority that are ready to run.   All tasks whose priority is less than or equal to the specified time-slice priority are time-sliced.

The Solaris threads scheduler does not directly support time-slicing of threads but the threads library contains the functionality necessary for time-slicing to be implemented in the Ada runtime layer.   Time-slicing can be accomplished by attaching a clock interrupt handler with the timer set to the time slice interval. When the clock interrupt handler is executed, it calls *thr_yield*, which preempts the executing task if another thread of the same or higher priority is ready to execute.

13. Debugging

The SPARCompiler Ada multithread (MT) debugger operates synchronously with the program. When a breakpoint is reached, all of the tasks in the program stop.   Similarly, when the user continues from a breakpoint, all of the executing tasks continue. Between the time the debugger stops and restarts a program, the operating system may reschedule the pool of LWPs onto the processors.

The MT debugger   recognizes and processes all of the non-threaded debugging commands and provides new information about threads.   Furthermore, the list tasks command (*lt*) has been extended to display the *thread_id* of the thread that corresponds to the Ada task. While debugging, it is possible to stop a program while it is executing one of the idle threads created for the threads library. The *lt* command identifies these threads as "non-Ada tasks." At this point it is possible to change context to an Ada task using the *task* command.

When you select a different task in the debugger, it may not be possible for the debugger to determine all values in the registers.   This is because not all the register values are saved and restored by context switches at the Ada or at the threads level.

Typically, the debugger intercepts all signals and sends them to the program. However, the threads library uses several signals: SIGALRM, SIGLWP, and SIGWAITIN; therefore, the multithread debugger ignores these signals.

To support debugging in the Solaris multithread architecture, changes are made at the system level by adding extensions to the */proc* file system. */proc* provides debugger access at the LWP level but not at the threads level.   A separate interface was created for debugger control of threads, referred to as *thread_db*. The *thread_db* interface was originally designed for dbx debugging and was found to be inadequate for the Ada debugger. As a result, the Ada debugger must currently rely on internal knowledge of threads data structures to support debugging of threaded programs.   Work is progressing on a new threads debugger interface which is language independent. This interface will support services such as getting the current thread id, reading and writing general and floating point registers for a thread id, and determining the current state and attributes of a thread.

In addition to the use of the standardized debugger interface when it becomes available, future SPARCompiler Ada debugger work includes an asynchronous debugger, allowing the user to start and stop tasks individually; future commands will also provide more information about the LWPs and threads in the process.

14. Statistical Profiler

The SPARCompiler Ada toolset contains a statistical profiler, which collects and displays information about the CPU usage of a program. This tool is very valuable for determining which routines consume the highest CPU usage, and for determining how many times a routine is called and the average number of milliseconds spent in the routine per call. At execution time, the Ada runtime startup code attaches a signal handler for program exit, then calls the Solaris system call *profil*, which provides kernel support for the collection of profiling data. *profil* works by examining the program counter (PC) for every clock tick and incrementing a counter for the code associated with the PC. When the program exits, the profiling exit signal handler is executed, it calls *profil* to stop profiling, then it writes the profiling data buffer information to a data file. The information in the profile data file can be interpreted and displayed after program execution completes, using the Solaris *prof* utility or the SPARCompiler Ada *a.prof* command which understands Ada subprogram naming conventions.

The Solaris multi-thread architecture provides one interval timer per LWP and the ability to enable profiling for each individual LWP using *profil*. A separate profile data buffer can be specified for each LWP, or a single profiling buffer can be shared by two or more LWPs to collect accumulated data. It is currently not possible to collect profile data on a per-thread basis unless each thread is created bound and profiling is enabled for each of the LWPs. This requires calling *profil* for each of the LWPs. It is difficult to collect profiling data for unbound threads because the threads library can create LWPs as needed to avoid deadlock, unknown to the application or Ada runtime. In this scenario there is no way for the Ada runtime to know when a new LWP is created so it cannot call *profil* to enable profiling for that LWP. Profiling models which provide a profile buffer per thread have an unacceptably high overhead. Alternate profiling models are currently being investigated that would allow profiling data to be collected for bound and unbound threads.

15. Libraries and Bindings

Interfacing to routines in libraries require care in a threaded environment. An application cannot arbitrarily enter non-threaded code, such as an mt-unsafe function in a library. An mt-safe routine is one which executes correctly in parallel. Due to problems with error codes, only the main thread can call unsafe code. Library routines traditionally return an error code allocated in static, global storage. This model does not work in a multithreaded environment, where each thread has its own error variable allocated and managed in per-thread storage via thread specific data (TSD). It is possible to call mt-unsafe routines, if access to the routines is synchronized and if the synchronized protection includes access to implicit elements of the interface, such as error code globals.

Many of the commonly used system libraries have been made mt-safe. The current list of Solaris mt-safe libraries includes: libc, libm, libw, libintl, libmalloc, libmapmalloc, and libnsl (TLI interface portion). Many other libraries such as networking libraries and windows libraries are currently being modified to be mt-safe. Due to the current lack of mt-safe X and XView libraries, the SPARCompiler Ada/XView binding does not currently work with the threaded runtime, but the use of synchronization methods is being evaluated.

16. Testing

Ada proved to be extremely valuable in testing early versions of the Solaris threads library, due to the large number of existing Ada benchmarks, tests, and applications which take advantage of architecture parallelism when using Ada tasks. C applications, on the other hand, must be modified considerably to take advantage of the threads model, usually requiring a complete redesign of the software. Existing Ada test suites such as ACVC, CAMP, PIWG, and so forth required only recompilation and relinking to run on the Solaris multithreaded architecture.

It should be noted that an Ada program with tasks that executes correctly on a single processor system is not guaranteed to execute correctly when the tasks run in parallel on a multiprocessor system. The application must be careful not to use task priorities to serialize execution. When executing on a single CPU, task priorities can be used to guarantee the order of execution, but this does not hold true on an MP where multiple tasks can execute simultaneously. Similarly, disabling preemption cannot be used as a means of serializing execution for the same reasons.

17. Performance

Benchmarks such as PIWGs show slightly higher overhead in task creation and rendezvous times with the use of threads. For most applications, the small threads overhead is negligible on a single processor and is typically offset on multiprocessor systems by the huge performance gains which are possible due to the parallel execution of the Ada tasks. Solaris is designed to perform well on both multiprocessor and single processor systems. Because of its symmetric design, Solaris results in throughput increases proportional to the number of processors in the system. In some cases, it is even possible to see increased performance on a single processor system for applications which previously blocked on I/O or other system calls.

18. Ada 9X

Two of the major goals of Ada 9X are to provide additional functionality and performance improvements, especially in the area of real-time and parallel programming. In its efforts to meet the goals of real-time users, Ada 9X provides new language features which provide faster task synchronization and communication, as well as additional controls for task scheduling, priorities, and entry selection.

The remainder of this paper discusses Ada 9X features which have an impact on the Ada runtime system implemented with Solaris Threads. Compiler and linker impact of Ada 9X features is outside the scope of this paper, which will focus on the feasibility of implementing Ada 9X with a multithreaded operating system performing the scheduling and communication of Ada entities.

19. Protected Types

One of the weaknesses of Ada 83 is the lack of language support for asynchronous communication. Many types of applications require a lower level form of communication than the Ada 83 task rendezvous which provides synchronous communication. This has led to implementation of specific versions of asynchronous communication which are generally non-portable. The addition of the "protected type" in Ada 9X provides direct language support for asynchronous communication.

There are two basic components to protected types, protected operations and private data components.   Protected operations have exclusive access to the private data components and are locked while executing its operations. The lock can be read-write for protected procedures and protected entries, and write locked for protected functions. Each entry body has an "entry barrier". The caller of an entry is suspended if the barrier is false. Each entry has an entry queue for suspended callers. A common use of protected types is to define data which is shared between multiple tasks as private data components. The protected operations define the operations available for the shared data.

Protected types in Ada 9X are basically providing mutually exclusive access to shared data. Protected types can be used to support semaphores and mutexes, and to define critical regions and additional synchronization constructs. As such, the implementation of protected types using Solaris Threads, while not trival, is very straightforward and does not require extensions to existing threads facilities. The Ada runtime will require additional runtime data structures to maintain protected type information such as the state of the lock, a queue containing callers of the protected entry, and so forth. A conditional wait (*cond_wait*) can be used to implement the protected entry barriers. When the condition variable becomes true, the Ada runtime can acquire a mutex by calling *mutex_lock* to execute the protected entry body. The runtime must also change the priority of the task calling the protected operation to the ceiling priority of the protected object. On completion of the protected procedure or protected entry, the Ada runtime releases the mutex by calling *mutex_unlock* and resets the priority of the calling task to its original value.

20. Requeue

Another new feature of Ada 9X is the requeue statement, which is allowed in entry bodies and accept bodies. Each protected record entry has an associated queue. Tasks wait in the queue until the entry's barrier becomes true. The requeue statement allows the caller to return to the same queue, to a different entry queue of the same protected record, or to an entry of a different protected record. The advantage of the requeue statement is that it allows a task to be moved to another entry queue without being resumed and having to initiate another entry call.

Implementating a requeue operation to the same queue or to a different queue can be accomplished with the same threads services necessary for the implementation of protected types - condition variables and mutexes. The requeue operation to the same queue is not very difficult. It requires updating Ada runtime data structures containing entry queue information and modifications to task state data structures. Next the entry barrier, which is implemented as a condition variable, is evaluated to determine if the calling task can execute the entry. The priority of the task does not need to be modified and the mutex does not have to be reaquired. A requeue operation to a different entry is slightly more complicated. The Ada runtime must change the priority of the task calling the protected operation to the ceiling priority of the protected object and must acquire a mutex by calling *mutex_lock* to execute the protected entry body. The entry barrier is evaluated and the entry body executes if the entry barrier value is true, otherwise the calling task is put on the entry queue. On completion of the protected procedure or protected entry, the Ada runtime releases the mutex by calling *mutex_unlock* and resets the priority of the calling task to its original value.

21. Priorities and Scheduling

In Ada 9X, each task has a base priority which can be changed dynamically by the user. There is also an active priority associated with each task. The active priority may be increased by the runtime to perform certain tasking operations, such as a rendezvous. For each protected record there is a ceiling priority, which is the upper bound for the active priorities of tasks that may call protected operations of that protected record. Ada 9X also defines a range of interrupt priority levels, which are higher than the task priority levels.

In addition to the priority-based scheduling supported in Ada 83, Ada 9X allows implementations to define and support other scheduling policies. The real-time systems annex defines a priority-based scheduling policy based on a dispatching model. The task dispatching policy specifies rules which are configurable by the user, such as when tasks are inserted and deleted from the ready queues, and whether a task is inserted at the head or the tail of the queue for its active priority. A configuration pragma specifies the task dispatching policy.

Support for scheduling policies other than the current priority-based allocation is highly dependent on the underlying threads scheduling performed by the Solaris threads library. The Ada runtime does not maintain the ready, running, or blocked queues, this is all performed by the threads implementation. Support for alternative scheduling policies must be implemented in the threads layer.

Queue scheduling is distinct from task scheduling. The core Ada 9X language defines a FIFO queuing policy. In addition, the real-time annex supports a priority queuing policy and allows an implementation to define other entry queuing policies. An implementation defined queue policy must specify rules for entry queuing order, the choice among open alternatives of a selective wait statement, and the choice among open entries of a protected object.

The implementation of priority queuing requires priority based mutex and condition variables. These features are not currently supported in the Solaris 2 implementation of threads and will be required to implement these features for Ada 9X.

22. Asynchronous Transfer of Control

Asynchronous transfer of control is a very important feature in Ada 9X. Ada 83 supports limited asynchronous execution with the abort statement, but what is really needed is a way for an external event to cause a task to begin executing at a new point, without causing the task to abort or restart.

Ada 9X supports asynchronous execution with a select statement containing an abortable part and a triggering alternative. The abortable final part runs if none of the select alternatives is immediately selected. The select alternatives are not cancelled when the abortable final part begins; instead they remain pending. If one of them is selected before the final part completes, then the sequence of statements of the abortable final part is aborted, and an asynchronous transfer of control takes place to the sequence of statements of the selected alternative. If the abortable part completes before the select alternative, then the select alternative is abandoned. The select alternative can be a delay statement or an entry call.

For the Ada runtime, asynchronous transfer of control adds considerable overhead and complexity to the tasking mechanism. A detailed investigation of the implementation of this feature has not been completed, but preliminary investigations do not show this capability requiring new features or extensions to the Solaris Threads model.

23. Delays, Duration, and Time

New in Ada 9X is the delay-until statement. Rather than specifying a duration as in the Ada 83 delay statement, the user specifies a wake-up time. This feature allows a task to wake up at a specific interval, as opposed to the Ada 83 delay statement, which supports specification of a minimum interval.

Solaris Threads supports a conditional wait, *cond_timedwait*. When *cond_timedwait* is used the calling thread will not block past the time specified in the time parameter. The time parameter is an absolute time, accurate to nanoseconds. The delay-until statement specifies a time rather than a duration for its argument so it can be directly mapped to the *cond_timedwait* call.

The real-time annex specifies an additional time type, MONOTONIC.TIME which can represent a real-time clock with potentially finer granularity than the time-of-day clock associated with CALENDAR.TIME. Unlike CALENDAR.CLOCK, the MONOTONIC.CLOCK function returns a value guaranteed to be monotonically non-decreasing.

Previous timer resolution was supported only to the microsecond level. but with Solaris 2 there is support for high resolution timers nanosecond accuracy. Operations are provided for high resolution timer operations to get the system time, add, subtract and compare two high resolution times, and to convert high resolution time values to a variety of formats. These routines provide the accuracy necessary to implement MONOTONIC.TIME in Ada 9X.

24. Summary

In summary, Solaris threads provide an ideal platform for the implementation of an Ada runtime system. The Ada runtime can focus on the details of implementing Ada tasking operations such as task activation, rendezvous, and abort, and the Solaris multithreaded environment handles scheduling and communication on one or more processors. The existing SPARCompiler Ada 83 implementation fulfills time-critical requirements through the use of standard Ada, allowing very portable and maintainable code which runs efficiently on uniprocessor and multiprocessor systems. Preliminary investigations show Solaris threads contains support for the implementation of the "core" Ada 9X language but extensions and enhancements to the threads model and the threads scheduler are necessary to implement some features of the Ada 9X real-time annex.

REFERENCES

[1] M.L. Powell, S.R. Kleiman, S. Barton, D. Shah, D. Stein, M. Weeks. SunOS 5.0 *Multithread Architecture*, SunSoft White Paper, 1991.

[2] Atri Chatterjee, Jim Herriot. *Multithreading and Real-Time*, SunSoft. White Paper, 1991.

[3] Sun Microsystems Inc. *SunOS Multi-Thread Architecture*, Revision 1.1, August 22, 1990.

[4] Robert B.K. Dewar, Matthew Smosna. "Previewing SunSoft's Solaris," *UNIX Today!* October 28, 1991.

[5] Bill O. Gallmeister. "Reconciling UNIX, Ada, & Real-Time Processing," *Dr. Dobbs Journal*, June 1991.

[6] David Simpson. "Will the real-time UNIX please stand up?" *Systems Integration*, December 1989.

[7] Grady Booch. *Software Engineering with Ada*, The Benjamin/Cummings Publishing Company, Inc., 1983.

[8] S.Tucker Taft. "Ada 9X: A Technical Summary," *Communications of the ACM*, November 1992.

[9] Karen Sielski. "Implementing Ada Tasking in a Multiprocessing, Multithreaded UNIX Environment," TRI-Ada Conference Procedings, November 1992.

Ada: Towards Maturity
Ed. L. Collingbourne
IOS Press 1993

Towards Distributed Objects in Ada 9X

Anthony Gargaro
Computer Sciences Corporation, Moorestown, New Jersey, USA

Abstract. The Distributed Systems Annex of Ada 9X [1] supports dynamically bound remote subprogram calls. Such calls when combined with the language enhancements for object-oriented programming allow objects to be remotely accessible across a distributed system. This paper advances a technique for programming such objects to enhance component-based software engineering.

1. Introduction

Recent interest in component-based software engineering for life-cycle management has focused on object-like software components. This focus is motivated by expectations that object-oriented programming provides an improved discipline for applying a seamless integration and management approach to developing very large software applications (sometimes termed *megamodules* [2]). In many instances, a megamodule represents a distributed system of software components. Consequently, programming abstractions for megamodules should be object-oriented and adaptable to distributed systems.

Ideally, megamodules support the interaction of loosely coupled, distributed, concurrently executing components or modules. Such components are characterized by three boundaries [3]: the *abstraction boundary*, the *distribution boundary*, and the *synchronisation boundary*. When the abstraction and distribution boundaries overlap, the component is a potentially distributed component. While Ada 9X does not specify a linguistic construct to represent distributed components, the Ada 9X enhancements for objected-oriented programming [4], combined with the capability to call dynamically bound remote subprograms, allow the construction of *distributed objects*.

This paper summarizes the notion of distributed objects, the Ada 9X partition model for distributed systems, and the approach for calling dynamically bound remote subprograms. This summary is followed by the introduction of a technique for constructing distributed object types to facilitate the goal of component-based software engineering. In conclusion, a perspective of this technique is compared to alternative approaches for distributed programming.

2. Distributed Objects

The term *distributed objects* has been popularized to convey the property of using the *abstraction-based* and *object-oriented* programming paradigms in a distributed network environment [5]. In this enhanced paradigm the client-server role is developed at a finer level of abstraction to achieve a more dynamic and transient computing model. The ability to call services of remotely located objects is an important requirement and is the origin for the terminology (since the actual object does not span multiple address spaces). Furthermore, this ability must be provided in a familiar and portable manner for both locally and remotely executed services.

In its simplest abstraction-based form, a distributed object may be viewed as an instance of an *abstract data type* whose associated services (operations) may be called by remote clients. Such objects may be replicated throughout a distributed systems environment to support highly parallel or fault-tolerant services to their clients. Typically the clients execute as components of a distributed system. The services are provided to clients using variations of *remote procedure calls*. All that is required to use the service is a reference to the object and the name of the service and associated parameter profile. Each object replica offers the same set of services; these services execute in the context of the environment where the object is created. Unlike their non-distributed counterparts, this context maintains an independent state for each replica. Object services access data only in the same context as the object or in contexts that are shared among clients and objects. To ameliorate the increased cost of executing a service, clients need not wait for the service to complete. Moreover, there is no requirement to synchronise concurrent calls to services unless the calls are to the same object. When synchronisation is required, to avoid logical inconsistencies within the object, the object may enforce this control prior to executing the service.

Enhancing the abstraction-based form to an object-oriented form allows the services to more readily adapt to the context where the object is created so that the objects are not constrained by the limitations imposed by replication. The data encapsulated by the object may be extended, and the object's services modified accordingly, while retaining the identical calling specifications for clients. For example, objects may be created that adapt to varying levels of resource availability depending upon where the object is created. In this way, for example, a distributed system may be programmed to execute in different modes where mode changes need not be detected by the clients.

The notion of distributed objects assumes coordination and management of objects throughout the distributed system by some kind of *object broker* [6] or distribution agent. Objects register their availability through the broker which then allows clients to reference them in order to use their services. In addition, a network communication undercarriage is assumed that provides the necessary message transmissions to support the remote calls to these services.

In summary, the properties of distributed objects facilitate a programming paradigm that allows the object's reusable services (the abstraction boundary) to adapt to its context (the distribution boundary) and that promotes independent, potentially parallel, execution (the synchronization boundary).

3. Model for Distributing an Ada 9X Program

The Ada 9X model for programming distributed systems specifies a *partition* as the unit of distribution. The model borrows from the *virtual node* concept [7,8] and earlier work that developed the concept into a partition construct [9] and specifies a simple, consistent, and systematic approach towards composing distributed systems. Partitions comprise aggregations of library units that elaborate and execute independently using a distributed target execution environment. Typically, each partition corresponds to a single execution site where all its library units occupy the same logical address space. The principal interface between partitions is one or more package specifications.

Partitions may be either *active* or *passive*. An active partition comprises library units that reside and execute upon the same *processor module*. In contrast, library units constituting a passive partition reside at a *common address space module* that is accessible to the processor modules of different active partitions that reference them.

Partitions are specified subsequent to the compilation of their constituent library units. Programming cooperation among partitions is achieved through library level *preelaborable* packages that allow access to data and subprograms in different partitions to which these packages are explicitly *assigned*. These library packages are identified at compile-time by *categorization pragmas*. This maintains type safety and unit consistency across a distributed system, while avoiding the complexity of a distributed run-time system.

An active partition may name *shared passive packages* from passive partitions in its closure, thus referencing packages common to other partitions in the distributed system. Different active partitions (executing in separate processor modules) may reference the same data or execute subprograms from such packages.

Active partitions may call subprograms in other active partitions. Calls to subprograms in a different active partition are allowed only if the called subprogram is referenced (explicitly or implicitly) through a package that is compiled with the categorization pragma Remote_Call_Interface. An active partition must include a *remote call interface* (RCI) package in order to call a subprogram in a different partition. When an active partition calls such a subprogram, the call is termed a *remote subprogram call*. In addition, an *asynchronous remote procedure call* capability is provided to allow the client partition and the called remote procedure to execute independently once the call has been sent to the remote server partition.

While the categorization of packages must be specified at compile time, the actual assignment to partitions is achieved subsequently (e.g., at link time) and is not specified by the model. A program may be partitioned differently, but each partitioning must remain semantically consistent with a single partition program. Each RCI or shared passive package may be assigned to only a single partition; however more than one of these packages may be assigned to the same partition. All library units named in the closure of their context clauses are included in the partition.

Unlike RCI and shared passive packages, library units that are not so categorized are replicated in each partition; the state of these packages is maintained independently. However, since the partitioning rules require all parameter types of remotely callable subprogram to be declared in preelaborable packages, there can be no inconsistency in the operand matching rules of remote subprogram calls.

Finally, a Partition Communication Subsystem (PCS) is defined to achieve remote subprogram call communication using different message transfer protocols. The PCS is a layer of software specifying a common package interface (RPC_Support) to which remote subprogram call implementations must conform. This allows a PCS to be implemented independently of a specific Ada 9X compiler. The PCS connects the compiler-generated code to the appropriate network communication stack software.

3.1. Statically Bound Remote Subprogram Calls

Statically bound remote subprogram calls follow the remote procedure call semantics that have been codified for standardization [10]. For example, remote subprograms are executed with *at-most-once* semantics. A client partition may call a subprogram in a server partition if the subprogram is declared in the visible part of an RCI package (and that RCI package has been explicitly assigned to the server partition).

When compiling the specification of an RCI package, *calling stubs* are generated for each visible subprogram. Similarly, when compiling the body of an RCI package, *receiving stubs* are generated. The calling stub marshals the subprogram parameters into a data stream (using the attribute 'Write) to be delivered to the server partition (through the PCS) and waits for and unmarshals any output parameters, result, or exception. The receiving stub unmarshals the data stream (using the attribute 'Read) into subprogram parameters and calls the subprogram for execution. Upon completion it marshals the output parameters, result, or exception into a data stream to be returned (through the PCS) to the client partition.

The form of a statically bound remote subprogram call is as follows:

```
package Remote_Services is
  pragma Remote_Call_Interface;
  type Object_Type is ...
  procedure Opn (Object : Object_Type; ...);
  ...
end Remote_Services;

-- The RCI package body is included in the server partition.
with ...
package body Remote_Services is
  procedure Opn (Object : Object_Type; ...) is
  ...
end Remote_Services;

-- The object elaboration and remote call are included in the client partition.
with Remote_Services;
...
Obj : Remote_Services.Object_Type;
...
Remote_Services.Opn (Obj, ...);        -- remote call to server partition
```

Statically bound remote calls follow the normal visibility rules of Ada. A client partition must include the RCI package specification that declares the subprogram to be called. Consequently, such calls are limited to paradigms that are not dependent upon a dynamic execution environment, as binding to the called partition is achieved prior to partition elaboration. Furthermore, although support for distributed objects rely on statically bound calls (viz., to communicate with the object broker), such calls are not used to provide remote services since the object and its services are typically elaborated in different partitions (as shown above).

3.2. Dynamically Bound Remote Subprogram Calls

Dynamically bound subprogram calls are supported in Ada 9X. In a single partition program, such calls are achieved by dereferencing an access-to-subprogram type object to call the designated subprogram, or by *dispatching* on a class-wide type controlling operand of a primitive operation for the specific type. Two forms of dynamic binding are adapted for distributed systems using *remote access-to-subprograms types* and *remote access-to-class-wide limited private types*. An advantage of using these forms of dynamic binding is they relax the requirement (of statically bound calls) for the calling partition to name in its closure the packages that explicitly declare the remote subprograms. Partitions need only name the RCI package that includes the declaration of an appropriate *remote access type*.

The access-to-class-wide form is a more object-oriented approach to providing remote services and allows the object and its remotely callable services to be encapsulated in the same partition (enabling the abstraction and distribution boundaries to coincide). The remotely callable subprograms are specified as the primitive *abstract* operations of a *tagged limited private type* in a *declared-pure* package (a preelaborable package that is replicated identically in all referent partitions). In an

RCI package, a remote access type designating the corresponding class-wide type is declared. This type allows values of the remote access type to be dereferenced as the controlling operand of the primitive operations. These operations are the remote services of the distributed object when *overridden* in the partition where the object is elaborated. For each remote access type declared in the visible part of an RCI package, calling and receiving stubs are generated for each primitive (dispatching) operation of the designated type.

This form of a dynamically bound remote subprogram call is as follows:

```
-- Package included in client and server partitions.
package Remote_Types is
  pragma Pure;
  type Object_Type is tagged limited private;
  procedure Opn (Object : access Object_Type; ...)is < >;
private
  ...
end Remote_Types;

-- Package body included in object broker partition.
with Remote_Types;
package Object_Broker is
  pragma Remote_Call_Interface;
  type Ref_Object_Type is access all Remote_Types.Object_Type'Class;
  function Next return Ref_Object_Type;
  procedure Register (Object : Ref_Object_Type);
end Object_Broker;

-- Package included in object server partition.
with Remote_Types;
package Object_Server is
  type Remote_Type is new Remote_Types.Object_Type with ...
  -- override primitive operation of parent type
  procedure Opn (Object : access Remote_Type; ...);
end Object_Server;

with Object_Broker;
package body Object_Server is
  D_Obj : Remote_Type;            -- potentially distributed object
  procedure Opn (Object : access Remote_Type; ...)is ...
begin
  -- register object with object broker partition
  Object_Broker.Register (D_Obj'Access);
end Object_Server;

-- Reference to object included in object client partition.
with Remote_Types, Object_Broker;
  ...
  Ref_Obj : Object_Broker.Ref_Object_Type := Object_Broker.Next;
  ...
  Remote_Types.Opn(Ref_Obj, ...);        -- remote dispatching call
```

The utility of this form of dynamic binding is achieved when it is combined with a name server or object broker partition using statically bound remote subprogram calls. Typically, the object broker partition provides a repository of remote access values designating objects throughout the entire distributed system. These values are available to client partitions (e.g., as shown by the function *Next* in the above outline). Consequently, this form leads towards a discipline for programming distributed objects.

4. Distributed Objects in Ada 9X

The previous sections have alluded to three boundaries that are useful in characterising distributed objects. While the language does not specify explicit constructs for distributed objects, a programming paradigm for distributed objects using remote access types may be described informally in terms of these conceptual boundaries. It should be noted that the paradigm presents one particular view of these boundaries; other paradigms may present different views.

4.1. Abstraction Boundary

The primitive operations of a tagged limited private type are used to represent this boundary. The type and its operations are encapsulated in a declared-pure package that may be included in any partition. Because such packages do not have state, each partition may reference them as if only a single instance of the packages exist. This provides a semantically consistent context for the abstraction boundary common to all types in the *derivation class* of the tagged type independent of the partition where the derived type declaration is elaborated.

The type is limited private; consequently, all visible operations must be explicitly specified. When these operations are abstract (there is no absolute requirement for the operations to be abstract), the type may be used only as the parent of a derivation class of types. Thus, since an object may not be declared using the parent type, a derived type with overriding operations must be declared in the same context where the distributed object elaborates. Moreover, since the controlling operand of each operation must be an access value, every call is performed by dereferencing this access value. If the access value is of a class-wide type, then the call is dynamically bound through the normal dispatching mechanism for tagged types.

These rules (or restrictions) allow an abstraction boundary to be partition independent. If these restrictions were not imposed, then the freedom permitted a single partition program would introduce implementation complexities to maintain consistent state and to support implicit (uncontrolled) remote references resulting from a multiple partition program.

4.2. Distribution Boundary

The remote access-to-class-wide limited private type in the RCI package implicitly represents this boundary. Every partition, either acting as a client or server, must include an RCI package with such a type to allow remote calls to the operations of a distributed object. Since the primitive operations of the designated type may be called by dereferencing values of the remote access type, these operations may be called remotely for any object type *covered* by the designated type. As a consequence, the abstraction and distribution boundaries are said to coincide conceptually.

The coincidence of these boundaries is a distinctive property of a distributed object. All objects of types within the derivative class designated by a remote access type are distributed objects since they either inherit or override remotely callable operations. Additional operations (primitive or otherwise) declared for a derived type cannot be called remotely since their visibility is local to the partition as a consequence of the rules for composing partitions; in other words, these operations are not within the intersection of the two boundaries.

4.3. Synchronisation Boundary

For a distributed object, its synchronisation boundary does not overlap the abstraction and distribution boundaries. This reflects that synchronisation control is bounded by a partition and is consistent with an implicit tenet of the partition model that distributed execution and synchronised control are orthogonal. Attempting to synchronise control across a distributed system is possible, but increases implementation complexity and introduces semantic difficulties (and is one reason that remote rendezvous is not supported by the model).

Synchronised control of a distributed object requires that access to its operations be mediated through some well-defined protocol once the server partition has been reached where the object was elaborated. This is necessary to allow the reliable execution of remote subprogram calls from multiple client partitions to the same object. Such control may be considered a property of the derivative class; in other words, types within the same derivative class should synchronise their operations uniformly whenever concurrent calls may be executed.

Unless this uniformity is present, unexpected interference may result when calling operations that have been implemented using inherited operations (a style endemic to object-oriented programming). This condition is manifested when, for example, an overriding operation reuses the overridden (inherited) operation and both operations have provided for access synchronisation using the same operand. This results in a deadlock when the overridden operation is called and cannot complete because it is unable to synchronise; e.g., when access to the operand is prevented by the calling (overriding) operation.

A single synchronisation protocol for each remotely called subprogram of a distributed object's type is defined. The remote subprogram, by dereferencing a controlling operand of the object's type, provides the necessary abstraction to reach the partition where the object is elaborated. Whereupon, this subprogram synchronises access to the object before executing a local subprogram call that implements the service to be performed.

An outline of this protocol is as follows:

```
procedure Remote_Opn (Object : access Obj_Type; ...)is
-- synchronise access to object
begin
   Local_Opn (Obj_Type'Class(Object.all));        -- perform requested service
end Remote_Opn;
```

Since the operand to the remote operation is an access-to-class-wide value, the appropriate local operation may be called by dispatching on the dereferenced class-wide (converted) operand. Consequently, the need to specify dual dispatching operations (for each remotely callable subprogram of a distributed object) becomes apparent: one that dispatches as a result of executing the receiving stub and one that dispatches as a result of executing the body of the remotely called subprogram.

These dispatching operations are declared as primitive operations for the derived type of the distributed object as follows:

```
type Obj_Type is new Remote_Type ...
-- override abstract operation of parent type
procedure Remote_Opn (Object : access Obj_Type; ...);
-- implement actual operation for object
procedure Local_Opn (Object : Obj_Type; ...);
```

A reliable technique for incorporating synchronisation control is relatively straightforward since the distributed object must be of a type derived from a class-wide type. This allows the object type to be extended with a component of a type that performs the synchronising actions within its primitive operations. All that remains is to arrange for these synchronisation operations to be enforced systematically. This may be achieved through the use of a *controlled* type with an *access discriminant* [11], where the type of the discriminant designates the type of the object extension. The *initialization* and *finalization* operations for the controlled type simply call the appropriate primitive operations of the designated type which are (or may call) the synchronising operations. In this way, the necessary synchronisation protocol for the distributed object can be engaged by declaring an object of the controlled type in the body of the remotely callable subprogram for the distributed object using the distributed object's extension component as the discriminant constraint.

An abbreviated outline of this technique using a simple semaphore is as follows:

```
protected type Flag_Type is ...
-- protected type with P and V semaphore operations

type Control_Type (Opn : access Flag_Type) is new Limited_Controlled with null;

procedure Initialize (Object : in out Control_Type) is
begin
  Object.Opn.P;         -- wait on semaphore
end Initialize;

procedure Finalize (Object : in out Control_Type) is
begin
  Object.Opn.V;         -- release semaphore
end Finalize;

type Obj_Type is new Remote_Type with record
  Control : Flag_Type;   -- protected object
end record;

procedure Remote_Opn (Object : access Obj_Type; ...)is
  Synch : Control_Type(Object.Control'Access);
  -- initialization operation reserves object
begin
  ...
  -- finalization operation releases object
end Remote_Opn;
```

An advantage of the above technique is that when the subprogram completes, the finalization operation executes the required resynchronisation; e.g., release a resource previously reserved by a semaphore.

Frequently, synchronisation to an object's services must be coordinated by the partition where the object is created, rather than by the object itself (as in the previous case). For example, the local partition may restrict clients from calling object services because of the lack of adequate processing resources. In this case, the partition requires the capability to prevent (or block) the execution of these services. Typically this can be accomplished only by inhibiting the client from invoking a remote service. Once the remote service is called, its execution cannot be intercepted by the called partition. Therefore, the system must be programmed to notify the clients that the object is no longer available; this is an expensive and drastic approach. Alternatively, the previously described technique may be adapted to provide a straightforward solution.

In contrast to the example of synchronisation controlled through the object, control is only required prior to executing the service. This control must determine if the service may proceed or wait until permitted by the object manager in the partition. This is achieved by passing an additional parameter to the initialization operation of the controlled object, which in turn passes it to a protected component of the distributed object that performs the determination.

The protected component may be declared using a protected type that implements the necessary synchronisation as follows:

```
-- The types Service_Type and Mask_Type are assumed to provide an
-- abstraction In_Mask that determines if a given service is masked.
protected type Synchronise_Type is
  entry Enter (Service : Service_Type);
  procedure Set_Mask (Mask : Mask_Type);
private
  entry Wait_Service (Boolean)(Service  : Service_Type);
  Alternate : Boolean := True;
  Service_Mask : Mask_Type := Initial_Value;
end Synchronise_Type;

protected body Synchronise_Type is
  procedure Set_Mask (Mask : Mask_Type) is
  begin
        Service_Mask := Mask;
        Alternate := not Alternate;
  end Set_Mask;

  entry Enter (Service : Service_Type) when True is
  begin
        if In_Mask(Service) then
          requeue Wait_Service(not Alternate) with abort;
        end if;
  end Enter;

  entry Wait_Service(for I in Boolean) (Service : Service_Type)
        when I = Alternate is
  begin
        if In_Mask(Service) then
          requeue Wait_Service(not Alternate) with abort;
        end if;
  end Wait_Service;
end Synchronise_Type;
```

Two public protected operations are provided: *Enter* that is called by the initialization operation, and *Set_Mask* that is called by the object manager component for the partition. A remote service may proceed only if the service is not included in one of the masked services. If the service is masked, then it is queued waiting until the object manager changes the mask to allow the service to proceed. In the protected type, *requeue* statements and a private entry family are used to simplify its implementation. While waiting to proceed, a service alternates between two queues of the entry family. A property of the alternating queues is that only one family member has enqueued entries (except when executing the private entry, *Wait_Service*). This guarantees that the order of execution for multiple calls for the same service is maintained.

Using this protected type and the earlier outlines, an outline for the packaging of a distributed object may be completed as follows:

```
-- Additional discriminant allows the remotely called service
-- to be passed as a parameter for permission to proceed.
type Control_Type (Opn : access Synchronise_Type; Service : Service_Type)
        is new Limited_Controlled with null;

procedure Initialize (Object : in out Control_Type) is
begin
   Object.Opn.Enter(Object.Service);
end Initialize;

type Obj_Type is new Remote_Type with record
   Control : Synchronise_Type;    -- protected object
end record;

procedure Remote_Service (Object : access Obj_Type; ...) is
   -- it is assumed that This_Service identifies called operation
   Synchronise : Control_Type(Object.Control'Access, This_Service);
begin
   ...
end Remote_Service;

-- Object elaborated in server partition.
D_Object : Obj_Type;
...
-- Server partition masks operations for object.
D_Object.Control.Set_Mask(Operation_Mask);
```

This particular synchronisation control specification for a distributed object allows an object manager to selectively choose among the different distributed object types it makes available to client partitions by simply masking all or none of their corresponding remote services.

The above technique may be adapted to use class-wide operands for the access discriminant and generic derived tagged types to parameterise the object extension in order to select different synchronisation protocols for each distributed object type [12]. This adaptation facilitates developing reusable components for programming increasingly sophisticated paradigms. Reusable components can be expressed as distributed objects by programming the appropriate services and synchronisation for the partition in which they are elaborated.

5. Conclusions

The different forms of statically and dynamically bound remote calls provide users with capabilities to program paradigms suited to distributed execution with only a small decrease in the level of abstraction from that of a corresponding local subprogram call. Both of these forms may be combined with the option to call remote procedures asynchronously when increased parallelism is required. This allows programming paradigms to achieve functionality that is usually available only in special-purpose academically developed languages. For example, rather than include a specific linguistic construct to support claiming output parameters from asynchronous remote procedure calls, such as *Promises* [13], a comparable abstraction may be programmed that transforms a procedure with *in* and *out* mode parameters into a procedure with *in* mode parameters, one of which is an access-to-subprogram value that designates a Promises-like object [12].

The inability to create and replicate partitions dynamically has been identified as a potential handicap to achieving fault-tolerant and highly-parallel programming in Ada 9X. While distributed objects moderate this handicap to some degree, it is recognised that although the objects may be created dynamically using access types, their context must be established statically (typically using a generic form of an RCI package). The accommodation of dynamic partition replication requires introducing an additional linguistic construct that many perceive as conflicting with the original language design principles. However, translating an extra-lingual partition type to a conforming Ada 9X program is an area of continuing research [14]. This research may yield a viable option when explicitly controlling partition creation and replication in a more dynamic environment is necessary.

Recently reported academic work indicates an increasing interest in advancing support for distributed programming paradigms [15], and in adapting existing object-oriented languages for distributed parallel execution [16]. This work may be contrasted with the Ada 9X approach to evaluate its contribution to the state-of-the-practice.

In the former work, a key concept is to specify pattern-based abstractions that facilitate *multicasting* messages among distributed objects for their services in order to enhance reliability and increase performance. These abstractions are intended to be incorporated by *Actor-like* languages rather than to provide a complete programming language. An example of a processor pool is presented as a problem in which the pattern-based abstractions provide an elegant solution. While lacking the claimed efficiency of this solution, the distributed object approach may be used to implement an alternative, but less ambitious, solution [12].

In the latter work, linguistic extensions are provided to the C++ language to support object classes that may be located in disjoint address spaces. Two new class definitions allow the declaration of distributed objects whose member functions are called by other objects using asynchronous remote procedure calls. A *return-to-future* feature is provided to forward results to other object member functions or to the calling function. Unlike the services provided by distributed objects of Ada 9X, member functions enforce monitor-like synchronisation, and thus preclude the ability to execute concurrent service requests for an object.

The need to introduce a pragmatic approach towards distributed execution within a proven reliable programmatic context is essential for component-based software engineering. Industrial initiatives have recognised this need [6] and such initiatives provide a useful comparison with the approach presented in this paper. While remote procedure calls are commonly used in these initiatives [17], the integration of remote procedure calls into a paradigm for programming distributed objects appears to be a distinction of Ada 9X.

The paradigm exploits the progression of Ada from an abstraction-based language to a language that supports both object-oriented programming and distributed systems. In addition, it exemplifies the enriched capabilities of the language to develop reliable and reusable components for concurrent execution. Moreover, its implementation is achieved without requiring significant advances in the state of compiler or run-time system technology.

6. Acknowledgements

The material for this paper resulted from collaborating with Offer Pazy and S. Tucker Taft, as a consultant to Intermetrics Inc. (Cambridge, MA, USA) Mapping Revision Team, in developing the Ada 9X Distributed Systems Annex under contract F08635-90-C-0066.

References

[1]   Intermetrics, Inc. *Annotated Ada 9X Reference Manual Draft, Version 2.0* (March 1993).

[2]   G. Wiederhold *et al.*, Toward Megaprogramming, *Commun. ACM 35, 11* (November 1992).

[3]   P. Wegner, Concepts and Paradigms of Object-Oriented Programming, *ACM SIGPLAN OOPS Messenger 1, 1* (August 1990).

[4]   J. Barnes, *Introducing Ada 9X*, Office of the Under Secretary of Defense for Acquisition (February 1993).

[5]   SunSoft, Distributed Objects Everywhere, *Project DOE* (1991).

[6]   Object Management Group, *The Common Object Request Broker: Architecture and Specification*, Object Management Group (1992).

[7]   S. Goldsack, *et al.*, Ada for Distributed Systems - A Library of Virtual Nodes, *Proceedings of the Ada Europe International Conference*, Cambridge University Press (June 1987).

[8]   A. Hutcheon and A. Wellings, The Virtual Node Approach to Designing Distributed Ada Programs, *Ada User 9* (December 1988).

[9]   A. Gargaro *et al.*, Toward Supporting Distributed Systems in Ada 9X, *Proceedings of the Ada Europe International Conference*, Cambridge University Press (June 1990).

[10]   ISO/IEC JTC1/SC21/WG8, *Open System Interconnection - Remote Procedure Call Specification Part 1: Model, CD 11758-1.2* (September 1992).

[11]   R. Duff, *LSN-50: Language Study Note on Access Discriminants*, Intermetrics, Inc. (November 1992).

[12]   A. Gargaro, Towards Distributed Programming Paradigms in Ada 9X, *Proceedings of the Tenth Annual ACM DC SIGAda/NASA Washington Ada Symposium* (June 1993).

[13]   B. Liskov and L. Shrira, Promises: Linguistic Support for Efficient Asynchronous Procedure Calls in Distributed Systems, *ACM SIGPLAN'88 Conference on Programming Language Design and Implementation* (June 1998).

[14]   S. Goldsack *et al.*, Translating an AdaPT Partition to Ada 9X, *Proceedings of the 6th International Workshop on Real-Time Ada Issues*, ACM SIGAda Letters XIII, 2 (March/April 1993).

[15]   G. Agha and C. Callsen, ActorSpace: An Open Distributed Programmimg Paradigm, *ACM SIGPLAN Notices 28, 7* (July 1993).

[16]   A. Grimshaw, Easy-to-Use Object-Oriented Parallel Processing with Mentat, *IEEE Computer 26, 5* (May 1993).

[17]   Open Software Foundation, *Remote Procedure Call in a Distributed Computing Environment*, Open Software Foundation (August 1991).

Ada: Towards Maturity
Ed. L. Collingbourne
IOS Press 1993

Pragmatic Design with Ada

Caroline LANGENSIEPEN
Time High Data Ltd, Hawkstone, Sibthorpe, Notts NG23 5PN

Abstract This paper examines some of the problems associated with the design and implementation of large real-time systems in Ada. Methods for reducing these problems are described, including the identification of patterns within the behaviour of the system leading to the use of standardised patterns for the structure of the solutions. Case studies from real-life projects are used to illustrate these ideas.

1. Introduction

Ada is normally considered the language of choice for large, complex real time systems, certainly if they have some safety, reliability or security requirement. Unfortunately such systems are prone to problems associated with their scale. This paper examines a few heuristics which may assist in solving these problems.

2. Problems in large projects

The main problem with large systems is communications. Other risks - timescales, underestimating effort, performance are true in all projects, but are compounded here by failures of communications. Typical aspects of the problem are:

• *Documentation*. On projects of more than 20 designers (particularly if they are working at geographically separated sites), design requires documentation standards for internal technical notes, codes of practice, formal reviews, reissue of notes etc. So any design change has significant overheads.

• *Team Consistency*. Because Ada has only been in use for a relatively short time on large projects, the staff experience will be very variable. There will be some staff with applications knowledge but little Ada. They will use a style they know, no matter that it may be inappropriate to the overall scale of the system. Some will be Ada experts but with little experience of the application. They will use sophisticated constructs which are hard to understand.

• *Solving the Wrong Problem*. In the past, the main problem on small projects was performance. This assumption has carried over to large projects, leading to an early concentration on performance at low level, determining data representations etc., even before the structure of the design has been established.

3. Heuristics

Some strategies to improve communication and aid the design process are now proposed. The larger the scale of the project, the earlier in the lifecycle the problems have to be attacked and strategies set in place, since it becomes very difficult to adopt them later.

4. Object Oriented Design and Firewalling

Object Oriented Design (OOD) is a good technique to apply on large projects. The main reasons are its ability to allow the isolation of problems, encapsulation of data, and firewalling risk - in other words, to ensure the right level of communication between applications. Its advertised features of maximising reuse, inheritance etc are of much less interest to the manager of a particular project unless the features enable him to reduce his cost to completion - the ability to reuse the code developed for one project on another cut no ice if the first project gains no direct financial benefit from it.

In any case, Ada is not really an OOD language, but the package structure enables Abstract Data Types (ADTs), Abstract State Machines (ASMs) etc to be cleanly built. Its lack of an inheritance capability seems not to be be a problem, as in the situations where it is used, there does not seem to be that much need for it. Large systems tend to be wide rather than deep - ie there are very few layers of specialisation on any class, but there may be very many classes.

If one has a very wide staff profile of experience, then OOD allows one to set novices to work in areas of low risk, and be confident that they cannot harm those areas of high risk. Areas where application knowledge is most important can be isolated from those "general software" areas - giving the former to applications experts and the latter to Ada experts.

It is often worth providing an interface package to an area of functionality to be used by all other clients, even if they could legitimately get in at a lower level. This firewalling ensures that if that functionality moves to another processor, then only the interface package body changes, to make VME calls, RPCs across Ethernet etc. Of course, the decision where to place these potential hardware boundaries depends on the data bandwidth of the boundary as well as its level of abstraction. This may seem obvious, but staff with experience only of small projects often do not consider the changes that might have to occur to the architecture of a large system. It is the capability to handle such changes that have to be built into the design methodology as well as the design itself, since the maintenance period on such a system could be up to 15 years.

In addition, when (not if) initial performance is much lower than required, individual areas can be "tuned" without impacting the rest of the system. Of course, if the system was designed without regard to the overall constraints of the hardware and primary customer requirements, then tuning will not be enough, but a "reasonable" design will benefit from the encapsulation first, and then worrying about performance later. The benefits gained by easier testing and integration outweigh the overheads particularly for very large systems.

5. Constructive Structural Distortion

"Lapses from purity" may be necessary in an otherwise object based design for practical and political reasons. Practically, there may be some aspects of the system which are too large and complex to allow the individual classes to deal with. Normally such functionality occurs at the periphery of the system - where the abstractions within it collide with the constraints of the user or devices attached. For example, the human computer interface (HCI) where driving the display devices may be too complex and device dependent for the individual classes to use. This is one area where tuning is almost inevitable, and since it is more likely that the tuning will be needed for HCI in general rather than the display of one class in particular, then this area should be isolated - even if its relationship with the rest of the system is now somewhat distorted.

Politically, it may be necessary to abstract on the basis of customer requirements rather than what seem the "best" boundaries for implementation. Use of the client view rather than the designer view can be beneficial because customers can see their prime functionality in the design, requirements traceability becomes easier and the inevitable specification changes tend to be more isolated, since they occur within the boundaries as seen by the customer.

Although the stability of the "Problem Domain Component" of design has been noted elsewhere (eg. by Coad and Yourdon [1]), the importance of ensuring that the design of this component closely maps to the customer view has not been stressed. Improving requirements traceability aids system integration, testing and acceptance, since these final critical stages of the system life-cycle are strongly tied to the requirements matrix, which is the formal way in which the customer communicates his needs to the designers.

6. Conventions and Nomenclature

One of the most cost-effective ways of improving communications is by establishing conventions early on. Most projects have standards for the diagrams, documents and file names. However, these will not tend to address the semantic meaning involved in the names of packages, operations and variables. More relevant is to set up a dictionary of terms, preferably taken from the problem space, which are used in a consistent way throughout the project. If the applications experts and the customer invariably refer to some concept via an abbreviated name, then that is the name that should be used throughout the design - for example 'package RNSH1C' rather than 'package Sub_Harpoon' in a Naval simulation.

Conventions for names, particularly of operations, ensure that clients know what they are getting when they try to use an offered service. A typical convention might standardise the meanings of the container class names eg Set, Queue, List, Stack, and the operation names eg Initialise, Shutdown, Add, Remove, Get, Put, Update. Where additional semantics are involved, the names should show additional sophistication. For example, Database_Set.Add (The_Item) is a simple addition of a new item to a container class, whereas Events_Set.Register (The_Event) will not only add the Event to the container class, but will do something else such as raising an alarm.

7. Don't Panic about Tasks

The risks of early concentration on task removal and other implementation details at the expense of a clean structural design are compounded by the effects of the staff profile. Experienced Ada users from non-real time backgrounds will liberally use tasks, even when no actual parallelism exists. Their software will work but it won't "perform" - that is achieve its response target or processing budget. Domain experts (who are often very wary of overheads) will be niggardly with tasks, trying to get away with a cyclic behaviour even when truly asychronous events are occuring - then using machine code or just faster cycles to improve their runtime response. This code may go quickly, but getting it to work is difficult.

To achieve consistency of style, use of tasking to desynchronise large areas of functionality should be encouraged, but further down within an application, designers must question whether additional parallelism or desynchronisation is really necessary. Performance of a

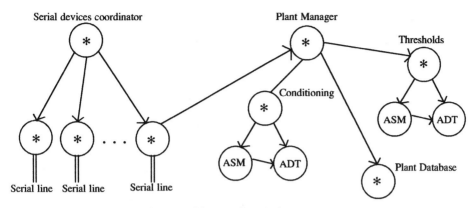

Figure 1 - Plant signal monitoring

system will not benefit from more tasks than there are processors or independent parallel i/o devices, but at the early stages of design there is no point worrying about them too much. If the task entry points are hidden behind a procedural interface, then from experience it seems to be comparatively simple to remove them at a later stage and by using the scenarios relating to the primary functionality, designers can easily count context switches, and test their design at each stage of iteration.

Consider a section of a project required to monitor a large number of plant variables via serial devices. Each of these plant signals requires conditioning (performing mathematical transformations upon it), testing against a set of threshold values, and recording the value of the signal in a database. The resultant design will therefore be based on operations on individual signals. Moreover, because the databases associated with the thresholds and treatments are also quite complex, the design protects them against concurrent access by their own tasking interface. A typical structural design for this is shown in figure 1.

By doing a simple count of context switches during the scenario of receiving a signal, processing and recording it, it soon becomes apparent that the tasking interfaces (as indicated by * in the diagram) would require many thousands of context switches a second for a typical large industrial application.. Yet the only really necessary tasks were those due to the true parallelism provided by the serial lines, a controller to initiate and query the states of the cards on these lines, and a tasking interface to ensure that external queries on the database would not clash with writes to it.

This removes the need for tasks in the areas of the conditioning, thresholds and database storage, leaving only one in the Plant Manager. Moreover, in the real situation from which this example was taken, the signals were received in groups of up to 256 per serial line interrupt, and by exporting a service that worked on the granularity of the hardware (ie the group of signals) rather than just a single signal, the switches were reduced still further. Context switches were reduced by a factor of 100, and this was achieved with no structural changes to the design and the provision of only a single extra exported operation in the Plant Manager. If the design had been started with the premise of using minimal tasks, then it is likely that the structure would never have been exposed - resulting in something very hard to test and maintain.

8. Find Patterns and Reuse them

Because of the 'width' of the large systems Ada tends to be used on, reuse of code tends to be minimal. Apart from using the same trivial set or queue construct, there is not much that be

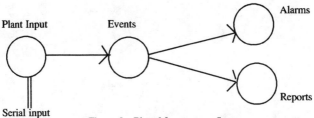

Serial input
Figure 2 - Plant Management System

reused from one application domain to another. Reuse of design also tends to be minimal unless obvious variants are being built. Reuse of 'meta-design' (that is, the principles and patterns used within the design) is possible and worthwhile.

Finding patterns in the problems and reusing the same structures of solutions in different areas helps in two ways. Once a solution has been found, finding the same pattern in the problem space of another application means the solution can just be ported. And using the same pattern (assisted by consistency of package and operation names) means that a maintainer can recognise it elsewhere and reduce his learning curve when looking at an unfamiliar area of software. The communications throughout the project are improved - everyone is talking 'the same language' .

8.1 Patterns in the Large

The first pattern to look for is the overall shape of the system to be developed. Three real-life problems will be considered as examples

a) Plant Management and Monitoring
This very large project for the monitoring of an industrial plant consists fundamentally of a set of serial devices (as described earlier), writing the status of the plant to a database, causing events to be generated if significant changes of state occur. The events and associated complex logic trees give rise to consequential actions - alarms are raised and reports may be generated (figure 2). The structure is very encapsulated, with each application area performing its functionality and then triggering another area to perform its behaviour as if by a control flow.

b) Command Team Training Simulator
This large project, to train a submarine command team, consists of a simulated scenario of ocean and vehicles, sonar simulations which build their 'pictures of the world' based on this scenario, and a simulation control module which allows the instructors to modify the scenario and examine the states of the sonar simulations (figure 3). This structure is very layered, with

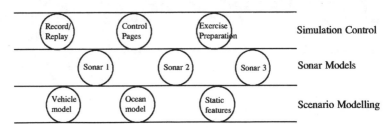

Figure 3 - Command Team Trainer

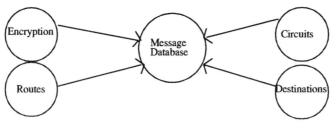

Figure 4 - Message Switch

all the simulations depending on the whole of the scenario, and the simulation control having a view of everything.

c) Message Switch
This smaller project, to receive, analyse, and route messages across a wide area network, consists essentially of the message database, with 'satellite' facilities serving this central concept. There may be facilities to set up routes, to engage and control encryption, to set up names of destinations etc, but all these are subordinate (figure 4). The structure is very centralised, with only one primary abstraction.

Note that nothing is 'purely' one shape. The Plant Management system might have a generalised layer for network communications, the message switch might have an event driven chain of side effects, but the primary shape is based on the primary functionality. Given these overall shapes, Ada will tend to suggest different development strategies:

a) There is not much commonality from one application area to another here, so given a definition of the very restricted interface provided to clients, each large area of functionality can be designed in parallel.
b)This structure means that every layer is very dependent on the layer(s) below it, so development has to be very bottom up, by defining the base scenario types (mass, time, length, acoustics etc) and the top scenario exports before then going on to work on the sonar simulation details.
c).In this situation, the message database exports must be very well developed first. Only then is it worth going on to develop the other lesser abstractions, since any change to the message will have an effect throughout the rest of the design.

8.2 Error Handling in the Large

One of the major problems with a large system is deciding on a consistent error and exception handling strategy that can be applied throughout the project. Of course, certain areas such as HCI have an obvious strategy, since errors in input are not really 'special' or exceptional, and so must be dealt with very locally. However, for the remainder of the system, the error handling will depend on the patterns seen so far.
Figure 5a occurs where the dependency is is wide, and cannot be segregated. For example, in the simulator described earlier the sonar depends on the ocean model, the vehicle model and practically every other element of the scenario. The simulator control has an equally wide dependance. Thus as soon as a fault occurs, say in the ocean modelling part of the scenario simulation, it affects all the sonars being simulated, and there is no point continuing. In that case, the fault may just as well be raised as an exception, and that allowed to propagate through the whole system.

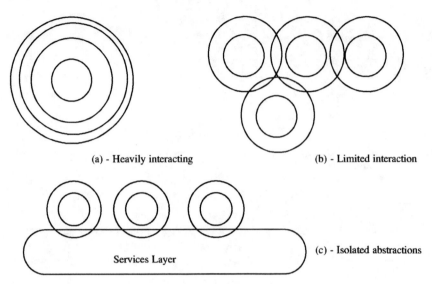

(a) - Heavily interacting   (b) - Limited interaction

Services Layer   (c) - Isolated abstractions

Figure 5 - Patterns in Dependency

Figure 5b has layers of functionality with high dependance, but then the outer layers of these interact with the outer layers of other applications. This is obviously true of the plant monitoring system, where there are layers within each application, but they only interact in a very limited way. The Shlaer-Mellor domain idea [2] can be mapped onto the layers in these applications. In this case, the existence of a fault deep within one domain should cause it to close down immediately, but a controlled closedown of the other domains can be performed since the interaction is so limited that the fault can be considered as localised.

Figure 5c takes this further, as in an ambulance command and control system. In these situations there may be some common layer, but a fault in one area need not impact another. Individual objects can be considered as isolated rather than the classes or class categories.This differs from cases like the plant input monitoring system shown earlier, where the signals are generated by common hardware in groups, and so cannot safely be considered as isolated. However, the incident in an ambulance command/control system is independent of other incidents. Allowing the fault to be isolated to the incident in which it occurred, and tripping out to manual only on that incident, ensures that the rest of the system can continue to function. In these safety related cases, losing the whole system due to a fault in a single object and forcing it to go to wholly manual operation reduces safety rather than improving it.

Later it will be seen where these layers can be considered to interact, and therefore where any exception handlers should occur.

8.3 Patterns in the Medium Scale

The patterns used in the medium scale tend to depend on their position in the application. At the periphery of a system, where the system interacts with humans or disc/tape devices, the behaviour is very different to that of the applications surrounded by other parts of the system.

a) Puppet Masters
Where the system meets the outside world, it has to translate commands from a generalised, non-abstracted form (eg keyboard input) into operations on the abstractions on the system. The knowledge of the abstractions contained in the semantics of the keyboard input has to be

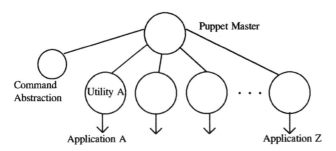

Figure 6 - the Puppet Master

converted into operations specifically acting on those abstractions. Thus the form tends to be of a transaction centre (a class utility) which accesses the generalised input/output (probably through additional layers of refinement and abstraction) and an associated ADT which expresses the final abstraction of the command or query (figure 6).

This transaction centre acts as a 'puppet master' pulling the strings of all the applications in the system as a result of the command. The ADT contains the semantics of the command, distilled away from the syntax or rules associated with the format of the interface. For an HCI layer which performs queries and commands on various applications, the ADT would express a verb (modify,delete), a subject (class name + id/name of object instance), and adjectives (attributes to modify). This ensures that whether the input is via a WIMP, preset hard keys, or standard keyed text, the abstracted command is the same. Below the puppet master, there are agent utilities which can interpret the adjectives to ensure correct parametrisation of the final call to the application. This structure ensures that not too much knowledge is forced up to the transaction centre, and the layers protect it against change, since the most likely change is in the parametrisation of specific operations on an application.

Another example of this is where a system has to have an associated simulator. Here, a text-based script is analysed and converted into script commands, which are then applied to various application areas. The advantage of this method is that the basic system can be written without worrying too much about the simulator. The simulator -specific functionality in the applications can be 'bolted on' as separate sub-packages within the top layer of each application. On top of all this sits the 'Script Puppet Master' which uses the script to run the applications by actioning their normal exported interfaces plus the new specific functionality.

A similar construct to this is known as the "Notifier" in SunView. The important point is not that this construct is new, but to recognise where it has to be created and used.

b) Managers
The most fundamental structure that is of use to a large system is that of an abstraction represented by an ADT and a container class to store instances of this abstraction. There is nothing going on but the addition and removal of various items from the container, and the examination and modification of their attributes.

Most situations in large real-time systems are more complicated than this. There may be side effects which have to be ensured, perhaps as a result of addition or removal of items from the container; multiple containers; state machines. A Manager is required to coordinate this complexity (figure 7).

The Manager, which has no specific abstraction, and no major local state, can ensure that concurrent access is controlled, and allow one to use a standard single-client version of the container class. As a finite state machine, it ensures that transient incomplete states are not

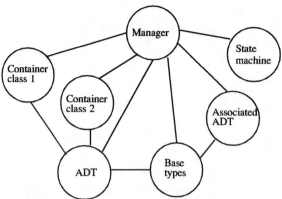

Figure 7 - the Manager

visible to clients. So, for example, if the generation of a new alarm must always be accompanied by the sounding of an audible annunciator, the manager ensures that it occurs. The manager also allows resistance to change. New hardware may allow the actual annunciator device state to be interrogated. When that occurs, the annunciator attribute associated with a particular alarm becomes redundant. By using a manager as the repository for this 'knowledge' of alarms, and annunciators, clients are unaffected when this change occurs.

It is also at this Manager level that any exception handling should occur, since the Manager can "interpret" the exception into a useful fault report. This limits the numbers of exception handlers required.

The concept of a Manager is very amenable to scaling. If a design starts off with a manager coordinating containers relating to separate classes, and then it is found that there is additional functionality (side effects, state machines) associated with these classes, then they can be hidden by another layer of managers. Note that this is not necessary if all one is doing is adding additional attributes to be recorded, modified, retrieved for an abstraction. Managers are needed to provide intelligence, to understand what needs to be done in addition to the simple change of an attribute. The question to be asked here is 'what is the added value?'. If a manager is not adding any additional meaning to what is going on in the container class or ADT, then it is not necessary.

Another advantage of the Manager structure is the ability to abstract away the 'real-time' behaviour of the system. In many large systems there is a substantial amount of off-line setting up of databases, which are then used online. For example, in a Sonar simulator, a complex mathematical model of the Ocean has to be run offline, and the results loaded to the online system for use during training. The offline and online systems must use the same ADT and possibly the same container class.

However, in the online system, there will be additional behaviour associated with these abstractions. If the ADT was maintained separately for both systems, there is a risk that they might get out of step, and the offline generated database would be incompatible with the online. If all offline facilities were available online, there is the danger that a future maintainer might accidentally build an application which used an illegal or inappropriate operation. However, by ensuring that all clients use the Manager interface, then safety is preserved, and the offline system can simply be built without the manager, to allow access to the full functionality to create the objects, but with no need to perform the online behaviour associated with the object.

c) Traffic Lights
Once a basic structural design is in place, the design has to start taking account of optimisation.

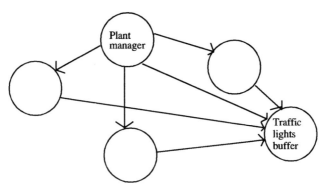

Figure 8 - the Traffic Lights Buffer

This is not searching for every last microsecond, which is not cost-effective on a large project, but performing optimisation in the large. Although the 'pure' design works in single entities, the hardware may work in particular aggregates, or it may be acceptable to run some things cyclically, if the loss of the last cycles information is acceptable on system failure. For example, the plant input system described earlier was optimised to handle a group of signals at a time, since that is the way the hardware provides them. Each signal may give rise an event, or generate a report, or may have to be passed on to another machine. If these are done individually, they would also slug performance. So the concept of a 'traffic lights' buffer is required (figure 8).

In order to ensure causality, all the actions resulting from a particular set of signals should be performed at the same granularity. If the report generation went on for each signal, while the events were buffered on some arbitrary basis, and the whole set of signals were not recorded until later, then the audit trail relating input and output actions could become fragmented. In addition, the report initiated by a signal might assume (legitimately) that the signal was already in the audit trail database when the report was being compiled, but in the above scenario this would not be true.

The traffic lights are 'set to red' while a group of signals are being processed. As a result of the process a number of different actions may be necessary, but instead of calling the appropriate application, the action waits at the traffic lights. When the group has been processed, the lights are 'set to green' and all the actions are performed, in the appropriate causal order, for the group. So in this case, the signals would all be recorded in the audit trail database before any events were registered or reports initiated. The release of this traffic is under the control of the manager processing the tranche of inputs, rather than the whim of the destination.

8.4 Patterns in the Small

Use of standardardised Sets, Queues etc. is commonplace, but these are so low level that the cost saving is small. More useful is to generate a house style for the specifications and bodies of project specific abstractions. For example, on the plant monitoring system discussed earlier, safety considerations and the possible fragmentation of the heap by use of 'new' declarations meant that true dynamic creation/deletion of objects was prohibited. Thus a 'Managed ADT' was required, which was a managed storage set masquerading as an ADT. By providing a standardised version of this common requirement, including its documentation, specific Initialise, Create, Destroy operations, and example implementations, one could be confident that the whole project would follow the same design for this component.

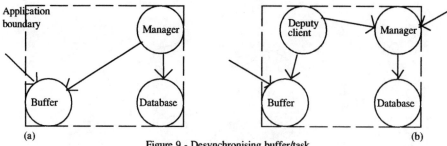

Figure 9 - Desynchronising buffer/task

Because of this prohibition on dynamic creation/deletion, another part of this system required a 'pseudo-dynamic' method of registering interest from various clients in Events. The events on which the resultant client action relied could be specified dynamically, but the client would not want to poll the Events database continually for anything of particular interest to it. The Events partition therefore exported a generic procedure which was instantiated by all potential clients.

Any partition could register itself as a client with Events on system initialisation and then register an interest in particular event ids. When an event changed state, the list of clients would be checked, and the generic procedure would action the procedure provided to it at instantiation as a formal parameter by each client. The advantage of this mechanism was that extra clients could be incorporated as the design evolved, and these clients could dynamically register and deregister interest in specific events without causing any dynamic space allocation/deallocation. This may be contrasted with the 'Phidippides' concept [3] which uses truly dynamic creation and deletion of tasks as messengers.

Other general requirements are the desynchronising buffer and desynchronising task. They are needed for clients whose main task is associated with interrupt generating hardware, for example the serial line devices mentioned earlier, or a system time facility which uses the clock interrupt, but 'kicks' applications to perform specific functionality at set times or intervals. Holding up these clients while a server performs some lengthy operation could cause them to miss their next interrupt.

The buffer concept is an obvious solution here, but the imprtant point is to place it within the domain boundary of the server application (figure 9a). In that way, any modification which might alter the way in which the server manager interacts with it has no impact outside the scope of the application. If the buffer were added as a separate design construct living somewhere between the clients and the server, then there would be overheads in documentation and retesting.

If an application has some operations which can be buffered, and some which have to be performed in the thread of the client, then the latter have to go directly throught the Manager, which, if it is providing concurrent access control, or atomicity of combinations of operations, will have a central task accepting their rendezvous. A single task cannot selectively accept client calls and take any buffered calls from the desynchronising buffer without polling or busy waiting This leads to the need for a desynchronising task, acting as a 'deputy client' (figure 9b). By preparing and disseminating standard versions of these constructs, the same structure could be reused easily.

9. Search for Misuse

In general, if one has an application area deep within a system, one would expect to see the following:

- 1 package for base types relating to attributes (the equivalent of 'Standard' for this application)
- A few true classes represented by ADT packages
- 1->a few container classes, the ASMs
- 0->a few utility packages, combining operations for the container classes
- 0->very few straight functions or side effects or state machines
- 1 Manager if >1 container class or side effects present.

In the above 'a few' means 2-3, but this is not a rule, just a measure for deciding whether the design needs looking at more closely to check its behaviour. For a transaction centre (as in the MMI or script case), expect to see a lot more utilities, but all with the same relationship to the central puppet master. If a partition has some critical response requirement, and a very limited number of clients, then one might expect to see utility or manager packages with operations "tuned" specifically to those clients. This is where pragmatism has to apply. A pure client-server architecture has servers who know nothing of their clients. But reality is never pure, and such compromises can improve performance out of proportion to their undesirable aspects.

If one sees more than one manager, then one worries about how atomicity of operations is being ensured, and concurrent access is being controlled. If there are a large number of classes exported by a package (rather than simple types exported by the 'Standard' package) then is there some confusion or amalgamation going on? A package may legitimately export more than one class if they are essentially different views of some underlying connecting abstraction, but would not expect to see that situation very often, and then only with a very few classes in a single package.

One must also look at how the behaviour will impact the clients. If an operation is exported which takes some time to perform, then can a client afford to be held up while it occurs? It is often forgotten that if a client cannot afford to be held up, then it is impacted by other clients who can, and which are waiting while some lengthy operations is performed within their thread of control. This is where desynchronising buffers or amalgamation of utility operations into the container classes for efficiency may be required.

10. Conclusion

The suggestions given above are not rules - they are simply ideas as to where to look for patterns in problems and solutions. The main purpose is to give some guidelines for improving communications and consistency, producing reasonable designs and recognising in time when the design is going wrong.

Acknowledgements

The author would like to thank Dr.R.J.Cant of Nottingham Trent University, Dr. P.R.Rees & D.Farquharson of Ferranti Industrial Systems, and T.Stuttard of Ferranti Simulation & Training for useful comments and suggestions.

References

[1] P.Coad, E.Yourdon, Object Oriented Design, Yourdon Press, 1991.
[2] S.Shlaer, S.J.Mellor, An Object-Oriented Approach to Domain Analysis, Software Engineering Notes, ACM Press, Vol. 14, No. 1, July 1989.
[3] A.Burns, Concurrent programming in Ada, Cambridge University Press, 1985

Ada: Towards Maturity
Ed. L. Collingbourne
IOS Press 1993

Experiences in Developing a Systems Trials Analysis Facility in Ada

Simon J. Barker

Electronic and Software Products, VSEL, Barrow-in-Furness, Cumbria

Abstract. This paper describes our on-going development of a System Trials Analysis Facility (STAF). The STAF is a stand alone system which accepts a range of data inputs from Combat System Equipments, which it synchronises and then analyses to provide graphical, geographical and tabular output. The analysed data is used to support the acceptance of a submarine combat systems. The STAF was developed for the MOD(PE).

1. Introduction

1.1 Overview

This paper will cover the following aspects of the development of the STAF :-

- use of Ada facilities to store variable amounts of data.

- use of Ada in a Motif environment to create a Graphical User Interface (GUI).

This is the first project to be developed by VSEL that uses both Ada and Motif. VSEL have already gained much experience in Ada with a number of accepted products since 1985 having been developed in Ada.

1.2 Development Environment

The Ada compiler used for this project is the Digital Ada compiler which VSEL consider to be the best compiler for a common host-target implementation on Digital equipment. The host-target is a Digital 4000 Model 60 Workstation with 80MB of memory and a selection of high capacity disk drives. A number of tape drives are also connected to the workstation to allow input from the Weapon Systems Equipments. The operating system is VMS.

To support the X-Window development, the VUIT tool supplied by Digital has been used. This enables a Motif conforming application to be created using a Motif tool kit which can then be integrated with an Ada application.

Some of the data to be analysed is supplied on DOS format 3.5 inch disks and these can be read directly at the workstation using the PCDISK facility of Digital's PATHWORKS tool.

1.3 System Design

The main constituents of the design of STAF are shown below :-

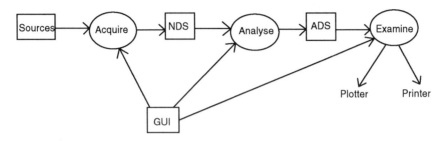

Figure 1 - STAF Design

Data is acquired from a number of sources and stored in the Normalised Data Store (NDS). This data is then analysed and the result of the analysis stored in the Analysed Data Store (ADS). The data in the ADS can then be examined for output to plotter or printer. The controlling process for these procedures is the Graphical User Interface (GUI).

This paper will address the design and implementation of the Normalised Data Store, Analysed Data Store, Graphical User Interface and Ada library software.

2. Normalised Data Store

2.1 Introduction

The STAF is required to consider over 350 different data parameters from its various data sources but the number of parameters for each analysis depends on the sources selected. Each parameter can have values for up to 16,200 time slices. A time slice is a time interval definable by the operator from 0.125 to 5 seconds. The number of time slices is also defined by the operator. Therefore a store is required that is very flexible and efficient in the way that it stores data and allows for fast retrieval.

The store is designed to contain upwards of 22Mb of data. The maximum size of objects is usually restricted by compilers (e.g to 64kb) therefore access types have to be used to create an object the size of the Normalised Data Store.

2.2 Implementation

The store is required to hold variable sizes of data, so it was decided to use access types in the implementation. There is no way of knowing how many of the parameters are going to be involved in an analysis so an array, indexed by parameter name, of pointers forms the basis of the store :-

```
type PARAMETER_POINTER_ARRAY_T is array (PARAMETER_NAME_T) of
     PARAMETER_ARRAY_POINTER_T;
```

Each pointer then points to an unconstrained array whose size is dictated by the number of time slices :-

> type NORMALISED_DATA_ARRAY_T is array (TIME_SLICE_NUMBER_T
>   range <>) of NORMALISED_DATA_RECORD_T;

Once the user has input the number of time slices, an array for a particular parameter can be initialised, using only the memory dictated by the number of time slices :-

> NORMALISED_DATA.PARAMETER_POINTER_ARRAY(PARAMETER_NAME).
>   DATA_ARRAY_POINTER :=
> new NORMALISED_DATA_ARRAY_T (1 .. MAXIMUM_TIME_SLICE_NUMBER);

Data is then acquired and used to fill up the arrays. Once all the data has been acquired, the arrays corresponding to each data parameter are written to disc and the memory deallocated.

The store is written as a package with the structure of the store in the package body. This is because the way the store is implemented is not required by a user of the store. A number of subprograms are then provided to allow the user to initialise the store, to read and write data and to write the store to disc.

3. Analysed Data Store

3.1 Introduction

The Normalised Data Store will usually contain a large amount data over a long time span. The user will normally wish to concentrate on a few parameters over a restricted time span. The Analysed Data Store is designed to store this subset of data. It also has to allow a sub-analysis to be created from the main analysis and graphs to be output to screen or plotter. The data itself is always displayed in tabular form, as shown below :-

Time	OS_HEADING	OS_DEPTH
12:40:00	34.2	21.8
12:40:10	34.2	21.8	← row
12:40:20	34.3	21.7
12:40:30	34.3	21.7
12:40:40	34.4	21.8
12:40:50	34.4	21.8	← cell

↑
column

Figure 2 - Analysed Data Store

The user can perform calculations across rows to determine errors and down columns to produce statistics. The analysis can be written to disc for merging with other analyses or further examination at a later date.

3.2 Implementation

Similar to the Normalised Data Store, the Analysed Data Store has to be flexible in the amount of data it holds. For this store, the number of data parameters is known, along with the number of time slices but the number of columns can be changed by the user if calculated columns are added. The columns are implemented as discriminated records whose parameter is the number of rows :-

```
type COLUMN_TYPE is array (MAX_ROWS_T range <>) of CELL_T;

type FLEXIBLE_COLUMN_TYPE_T (ROWS : MAX_ROWS_T := 1) is
    record
          ROW : COLUMN_TYPE(1 .. ROWS);
    end record;
```

The columns in the analysis are then declared using an unconstrained array of these discriminated records :-

```
type DATA_SECTION_T is array (MAX_COLUMNS_T range <>) of
    FLEXIBLE_COLUMN_TYPE_T;

type FLEXIBLE_DATA_SECTION_T (COLS : MAX_COLUMNS_T := 1) is
    record
          COL : DATA_SECTION_T (1 .. COLS);
    end record;
```

The Analysed Data Store allows columns to be added which are calculated from a pair of existing columns, e.g. the difference between two columns to determine a margin of error. The number of these calculated columns is variable so they are implemented using a linked list. Each entry in the linked list points to the flexible column type described above :-

```
type USER_DEFINED_COLUMNS_LINKED_LIST_T;
type USER_DEFINED_COLUMNS_POINTER_T is access
    USER_DEFINED_COLUMNS_LINKED_LIST_T;
type USER_DEFINED_COLUMNS_LINKED_LIST_T is
    record
          USER_DEFINED_DATA : FLEXIBLE_COLUMN_TYPE_T;
    end record;
```

A sub-analysis of the main analysis is implemented by storing which rows and columns are required for the sub-analysis rather than creating a new analysis file to contain the data. This also means that any data elements in an analysis which are modified are immediately seen in any sub-analysis or back to the main analysis.

As with the Normalised Data Store package, the implementation of the Analysed Data Store is hidden from the user.

4. Graphical User Interface

4.1 Introduction

The Graphical User Interface (GUI) follows the Motif standard for a window style interface as shown below :-

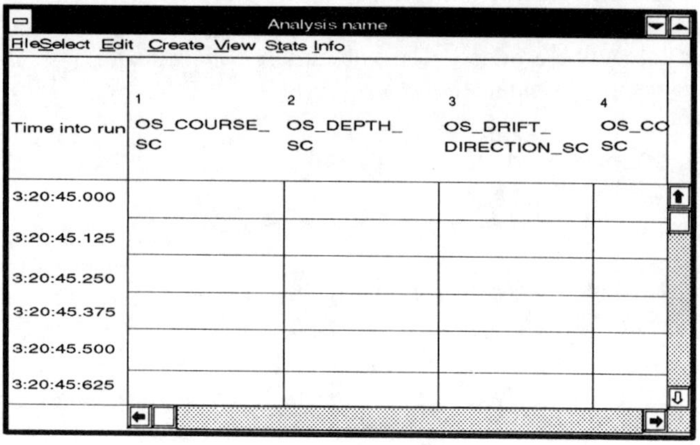

Figure 3 - Motif window

The windows are created using the VUIT tool supplied by Digital who also supply an Ada binding to Motif.

4.2 Implementation

The VUIT tool allows windows to be created with menus and the actions resulting from selecting items from these menus, therefore the creation of a prototype STAF was straightforward. This allowed the customer to be shown the interface at an early stage. The interface was an implementation of the User Manual which was written as soon as the requirements analysis had been completed. VUIT creates program stubs in Ada for any event associated with a window, e.g using a window button. The implementor then fills in the stub which, for example, calls an Ada procedure which creates the Normalised Data Store. For the drawing of graphs it has been necessary to call routines within the X library to provide the fine control for drawing lines etc.

The interface between Ada and Motif has proved to be a problem area. One reason is that Motif and the X library are implemented in the C language therefore frequent use has been made of access types and pointers. The following example shows how a string is obtained from a window :-

```
TEXT_PTR : MOTIF.STRING_TYPE; -- pointer to text in Motif

type ACCESS_STRING is access STRING (1 .. 10000); -- arbitrary length

function MOTIF_STRING_TO_ACCESS_STRING is new UNCHECKED_CONVERSION
```

(MOTIF.STRING_TYPE, ACCESS_STRING);
--converts Motif string pointer to a pointer to standard Ada string

begin

MOTIF.GET_STRING(RESULT => TEXT_PTR); -- get the value of Motif pointer

declare

S : STRING renames MOTIF_STRING_TO_ACCESS_STRING(TEXT_PTR).ALL;

The last line converts the Motif address using UNCHECKED_CONVERSION, then the ".ALL" suffix retrieves the data which is now accessible from the variable S as a standard Ada string. This procedure is typical of the mechanism to retrieve data from a window.

The use of pointers has resulted in conflict over accessing memory between the application and the operating system with a subsequent program crash which does not raise an Ada exception. A number of problems with the Ada Motif binding have been discovered and reported to Digital. This is thought to be one of the first projects to use Ada and Motif with VUIT therefore a number of problems could be expected.

5. Ada Library

5.1 Introduction

It was recognised that in the STAF, mathematical operations would be performed on items with the same dimensional unit, e.g. calculating the mean of a set of speeds and also a set of ranges. Therefore, it would be advantageous if the units could be implemented so that adding a speed to a range was indicated as illegal at compile time. For this, a library of Ada packages based on the SI system of units was devised.

5.2 Implementation

The implementation of each unit as a package is similar so the package for LENGTH will be considered here. A private type for DISTANCE is declared :-

type DISTANCE_T is private;

The Ada language will restrict operations to only assignment, equality and inequality. Therefore, the addition operation, for example, has to be defined :-

function "+"(L, R : in DISTANCE_T) return DISTANCE_T;

But there is no multiplication (or division) operation because the product of two dimensioned quantities has a different dimension. The package supplies routines for converting, e.g. a length in metres, to the type DISTANCE_T and in the reverse direction. Note that VSEL chose to implement LENGTH in metres but the user of the package does not need to know this, the implementation could have been in feet.

Once packages have been defined for LENGTH and TIME, then a package for VELOCITY can be defined which includes an operation for obtaining a velocity from a length and a time :-

function "/" (L : in DISTANCE_T; R : in DURATION) return SPEED_T;

Note that if the following are declared :-

A : DISTANCE_T;
B, C : SPEED_T;

Then this line will raise a compilation error because it is dimensionally incorrect:-

C := A + B;

If A, B and C had just been declared as INTEGER, for example, then the error might not have been detected until run time.

6. Conclusion

The STAF has proved to be a very valuable project for VSEL. The development of a GUI in the Ada language using Motif to run on a workstation will assist VSEL in future projects of this type. The creation of an Ada library of routines based on dimensioned quantities will also be available for re-use in future projects.

Ada: Towards Maturity
Ed. L. Collingbourne
IOS Press 1993

Ada 9X – Satisfying the Requirements

Bill TAYLOR

Transition Technology Limited, 96 Glanrhyd, Cwmbran, Gwent NP44 6TZ

Abstract. This paper compares the new capabilities of the Ada 9X language with
the original requirements for the language revision.

1. Introduction

The revision of the international Ada programming language standard [1], known as Ada
9X, has now reached the point where a draft Reference Manual has been submitted to
ISO/IEC JTC1/SC22, the subcommittee responsible for Programming Languages, for
registration as a *Committee Draft*. A revised draft is planned for September, for
consideration by the subcommittee. If acceptable, balloting on the draft will start in
October in parallel with an ANSI canvass. Following the inevitable changes to the
language (because of adverse comments during the ballot/canvass), a revised version will
be submitted to ISO/IEC JTC1, the parent body of SC22, to become a *Draft International
Standard*. A JTC1 ballot will be held, starting in about April 1994, in parallel with a
second ANSI canvass. This should be complete by October and a new standard available
in November 1994.

The revision process started in October 1988 with an open invitation to the world–wide
Ada community to send in *Revision Requests*. Over 770 were received ranging from
major changes to minor fixes, from the exciting to the bizarre. What was obvious was
that not all requests could be simultaneously satisfied and that even a compatible subset
would be beyond the scope of the proposed revision exercise – the changes were required
to have *minimum negative impact and maximum positive impact to the Ada Community*.

By the end of the first year, the Revision Requests and the set of Ada Commentaries
(approved interpretations of the 1983 standard) had been consolidated [2] into a set of 49
User Needs, 41 *Requirements* and 22 *Study Topics*. Study topics were for user needs
where it was unclear whether the benefits of making the change were worth the potential
costs. The Mapping/Revision Team were expected to address study topics with less
aggressive effort than the requirements. A full Rationale [3] was also produced, relating
the requirements and study topics to the Revision Requests, explaining why certain
Revision Requests had to be rejected and discussing alternative approaches for those
finally presented.

The next phase of the project was the *Mapping Phase*, proposing language changes to
satisfy the requirements and addressing as many of the study topics as was practicable in
the time available. This was followed by the *Revision Phase*, translating these changes
into revised wording in the Language Reference Manual. Successive version of a draft
manual were then produced. The information in this paper is based on Version 3.0 of the
Draft Reference Manual [4], produced in June 1993. A revised version is expected to be
submitted to SC22 in September.

1. Comparison of Proposed Changes with Requirements Document

Most but not all the User Needs in the Requirements Document have been addressed in the latest Reference Manual [4]. Many that are not included were addressed in earlier versions of the Mapping Document but removed following review comments that the impact of the change was not justified by the importance of the need.

The proposed Ada 9X language is analysed to see if each of the Requirements and Study Topics has been satisfied. The same section numbers are used as in the Requirements Document [2].

It should be noted that the Ada 9X definition is still changing – some of the proposed changes could be removed, and needs that have not been addressed could result in more change. This could occur before the standardisation process starts or as a result of comments received during the ANSI canvass or the ISO ballot.

2.   General Requirements

2.1. Presentation Requirements

Requirement R2.1–A(1) – Incorporate Approved Commentaries: Ada 9X shall incorporate the approved Ada Commentaries to the extent that they do not conflict with changes dictated by other requirements and to the extent that incorporation makes the wording of the standard clearer.

Discussion: The approved Commentaries have been incorporated by the ARG into the ACID (Ada Consolidated Issues Document). Similar changes have been considered during production of the Ada 9X Reference Manual.

Requirement R2.1–A(2) – Review Other Presentation Suggestions: Ada Commentaries in the *Presentation* class as well as the Revision Requests shall be examined for suggested wording improvements. Appropriate suggestions shall be incorporated into the revised standard.

Discussion: It is not currently clear how many such suggestions are appropriate.

Requirement R2.1–B(1) – Maintain Format of Existing Standard: the Ada 9X standard shall be similar in style and structure to the existing standard. Chapter and section headings and their order shall be retained to the largest extent possible. The presentation style shall also be retained.

Discussion: Chapter headings and their order have been retained (except that Chapter 9 is now called *Tasks and Synchronisation*), but are called *Sections*, to conform to ISO terminology. Section headings are mostly retained. The presentation style differs mainly because of ISO rules requiring use of "shall".

Requirement R2.1–C(1) – Machine–Readable Version of the Standard: A machine-readable version of the Ada 9X standard shall be made available using a widely supported formatting language.

Discussion: This is agreed in principle – the most appropriate formatting language is under consideration.

2.2. *Efficiency, Simplicity and Consistency*

Requirement R2.2–A(1) – Reduce Deterrents to Efficiency: Combinations of language features shall not incur compilation and execution costs (in time and space) that are significantly increase primarily because of extremely unlikely interactions with other language features.

Discussion: Two such rules are identified in the Requirements Document:

(a) *Access to Task Outside its Master*: in Ada 9X it is illegal or Program_Error is raised if a function with a result type with a task subcomponent returns a local variable. Note this rule is not upward compatible from Ada 83.

(b) *Null Ranges*: forcing S'Last to be the predecessor to S'First for a null range was considered but rejected as the (small) benefit did not justify the implementation/run-time cost.

Requirement R2.2–B(1) – Understandability: Rules that have proven to be confusing or error–prone to users shall be reviewed and eliminated when possible.

(a) *Elaboration Order*: two pragmas have been added: *Elaborate_All*, which is the transitive equivalent of pragma *Elaborate*; and *Elaborate_Body*, which forces the body to be elaborated immediately after the specification.

(b) *Later Declarative Items*: the distinction between basic declarative items and later declarative items has been removed.

(c) *Visibility of Literals and Operations*: In Ada 9X, character literals are visible everywhere; a *use–type* clause has been introduced to give visibility of primitive operators (but no other operations).

(d) *Obsolete Optional Bodies*: in Ada 9X, it is illegal to supply a body for a package that does not require one (but pragma *Elaborate_Body* forces a body to be required). Note this rule is not upward compatible from Ada 83.

(e) *Others clauses in Aggregates*: In Ada 9X, a named array aggregate can have an *others* choice, provided there is an applicable index constraint.

Requirement R2.2–C(1) – Minimise Special–Case Restrictions: To the extent consistent with Requirement R2.2–B(1), Ada 9X shall minimise exceptions to general rules specifying how language constructs interact. Special uses and combinations shall be eliminated.

Discussion: Thirteen such rules are identified in the Requirements Document:

(a) *Image and Value Attributes for Real Types*: in Ada 9X, these attributes are defined for all scalar types.

(b) *Exception Handlers in Accept Statements*: in Ada 9X, exception handlers are allowed in an accept body.

(c) *Range Attribute for Scalar Types*: in Ada 9X, the attribute *S'Range* can be used wherever *S'First .. S'Last* is allowed.

(d) *Permit Raise ... when <condition>*: this was originally proposed, but removed during the scope reduction activity.

(e) *Storage_Size for Task Objects*: in Ada 9X, *X'Storage_Size* can be defined for a task object *X*.

(f) *Explicit Type Conversions in Static Expressions*: in Ada 9X, the rules for static expressions have been generalised, including allowing type conversions, if the subtype–mark denotes a static scalar subtype.

(g) *Use of a Subprogram Name in its Specification*: in Ada 9X, a declaration is hidden from all visibility until the declaration is complete, thus allowing:

> **with** *Package_1;*
> **package** *Package_2* **is**
>   **procedure** *Procedure_1* **is new** *Package_1.Procedure_1;*
> **end** *Package_2;*

(h) *Default Names for Generic Formal Parameters*: no change has been made to satisfy this requirement.

(i) *Ability to Redefine "="*: in Ada 9X, explicit overloadings of "=" are permitted for any combination of parameter and result types. If the result type is not Boolean, "/=" can be explicitly overloaded.

(j) *Reading Out Parameters*: in Ada 9X, *out* parameters can be read.

(k) *Implicit Subtype Conversions*: in Ada 9X, subtype conversion (ie sliding) is allowed in all contexts except in a qualified–expression.

(l) *Negative Literals in Loops*: the following is legal in Ada 9X:

> **for** *N* **in** *–1 .. 1* **loop** ...

(m) *Naming Syntactic Items*: no change has been made to satisfy this requirement. The request was to allow if, case and select statements to be labelled and the label name used in the matching end.

2.3. Error Detection

Study Topic S2.3–A(1) – Improve Early Detection of Errors: If an implementation is able to detect that certain run–time program errors are present (eg that execution will necessarily be erroneous or that initialisation of a declared object will necessarily raise an exception), the implementation shall provide an option for rejecting the compilation (that is, not adding it to the program library). A similar option shall also be provided when a restriction associated with a pragma has been violated.

Discussion: Ada 9X implementations are free to provide such options.

Requirement R2.3–A(2) – Limit Consequences of Erroneous Executions: Run–time violations of language rules shall have narrowly defined consequences. Whenever practical, a violation shall result in the raising of an exception. When the raising of an exception is not practical, the possible consequences of the violation shall be few, confined to limited aspects of the computation state, and defined in the standard. This definition shall be in terms of those aspects of the computation state addressed elsewhere in the standard. To the extent possible, catastrophic consequences shall be excluded.

Discussion: In Ada 9X, the category of *Bounded Error* covers those cases where the possible behaviours are few. Most cases of Erroneous Execution fall into this category.

2.4. Controlling Implementation–Dependent Choices

Requirement R2.4–A(1) – Minimise Implementation–Dependences: Implementation dependences permitted in Ada 9X shall be justified by considerations of target architecture variations and different needs of applications. Ada 9X shall specify performance parameters and constraints affecting the use of critical constructs, although, since such constraints are typically application dependent, they should be specified in annexes.

Discussion: A number of implementation dependencies have been removed in Ada 9X, for example:

* rounding from real to integer is fully defined in Ada 9X (to be away from zero), thus *Integer (2.5)* is defined to be *3*.

Note that all such changes, while tightening the definition of the language, introduce a form of upward incompatibility from Ada 83 to Ada 9X

3.   Requirements for International Users

3.1. International Character Sets

Requirement R3.1–A(1) – Base Character Set: The Ada 9X type *Standard.Character* shall be based on ISO 8859, an 8–bit standard for character representation, in the same way that the Ada 83 character set is based on the ISO 646, a 7–bit standard.

Discussion: In Ada 9X, subtype *Standard.Character* will be based on the 8–bit ISO standard ISO 8859.

Requirement R3.1–A(2) – Extended Graphic Literals: Ada 9X shall permit the use of character and string literals containing non–English characters, including those from international character sets with more than 256 graphic symbols.

Discussion: Ada 9X will allow non–English characters, such as those in Latin–1, and those with 16–bit characters, via subtype *Standard.Wide_Character*.

Requirement R3.1–A(3) – Extended Character Set Support: Ada 9X shall provide input/output facilities and other operations for extended character sets (specifically, for international character sets with more than 256 graphic symbols). The operations shall be comparable to those provided for the current base character set.

Discussion: A separate version of Text_Io for Wide_Character is intended to be defined, called *Wide_Text_Io*.

Requirement R3.1–A(4) – Extended Comment Syntax: The use of international character sets (including those with more than 256 characters) shall continue to be permitted in comments in Ada 9X source code.

Discussion: In Ada 9X, any characters are allowed in comments.

Study Topic S3.1–A(5) – Extended Identifier Syntax: Ada 9X shall permit the use of extended character sets in identifiers while continuing to keep Ada's syntax and lexical rules independent of source code representation.

Discussion: Extended characters can be used in Ada identifiers.

4.   Support for Programming Paradigms

4.1.   Subprograms

Study Topic S4.1–A(1) – Subprograms as Objects: Ada 9X shall provide an easily implemented and efficient mechanism for dynamically selecting a subprogram that is to be called with a particular argument list; and a means of separating the set of subprograms that can be selected dynamically from the code that makes the selection.

Discussion: In Ada 9X, it is possible to define a type which can point to a subprogram, for example:

> **type** *Mess_Action* **is access procedure** *(M : Message);*

then given the following subprograms declarations:

> **procedure** *Store (M : Message);*
> **procedure** *Transmit (M : Message);*

the following are possible in Ada 9X:

> *Action : Message_Action := Store'Access;*
>
> *Action := Transmit'Access;*
>
> *Action ("Hello World")*

The attribute *'Access* is defined for any subprogram with a non–intrinsic calling convention. The variable *Action* can point to procedure *Store* or to procedure *Transmit* or to any other procedure with the same profile.

To ensure that taking *'Access* will never cause a dangling pointer, it is necessary to perform (compile–time) legality checks (called *accessibility* checks), to compare the life times of the type declaration and that of the subprogram.

Requirement R4.1–B(1) – Passing Subprograms as Parameters: Ada 9X shall provide a uniform means of passing subprograms as parameters to non–Ada procedures and functions.

Discussion: In Ada 9X, it is possible to define a type which can point to a subprogram, for example, given the declarations above, the following are possible in Ada 9X:

> **procedure** *Message_Handler (Action : Message_Action);*
>
> *Message_Handler (Store'Access);*

Message_Handler Transmit'Access);

Message_Handler (Action);

The procedure *Message_Handler* can be called with an actual parameter of *Store*, *Transmit*, or any procedure with the same profile (including the procedure designated by *Action*).

Requirement R4.1–B(2) – Pragma Interface: Ada 9X shall provide standard methods for specifying the link name of an externally defined subprogram and for specifying the parameter passing mechanism that is to be used. Other capabilities associated with pragma interface that are commonly provided by implementations today shall also be considered for standardisation.

Discussion: In Ada 9X, a new pragma (*Import*) has been defined which is the same as pragma *Interface* but allows a link name to be provided; no other capabilities have been added.

4.2. Storage Management

Requirement R4.2–A(1) – Allocation and Reclamation of Storage: Ada 9X shall allow an application to ensure that storage is allocated and reclaimed efficiently and predictably.

Discussion: Storage allocation/reclamation can be reliably controlled for user–defined types via the concept of *Storage_Pools* and the use of user–defined allocators.

The package *System.Storage_Pools* defines a controlled subtype (*Root_Storage_Pool*) with two abstract operations, *Allocate* and *Deallocate*.

A storage pool object must be declared of a subtype derived from *Root_Storage_Pool*.

The *Storage_Pool* attribute is used to associate an access type with the storage pool object, thus:

```
Pool_Object : Some_Storage_Pool_Type;

type T is access Designated_Subtype;
for T'Storage_Pool use Pool_Object;
```

Study topic S4.2–A(2) – Preservation of Abstraction: To the extent possible, Ada 9X shall meet Requirement R4.2–A(1) in a manner that allows storage allocation and reclamation to be controlled reliably for user–defined data types.

Discussion: User–defined assignment is available for types derived from *Finalization.Controlled*.

```
package Finalization is
    package Root_Controlled_Types is ...
    type Controlled is new Root_Controlled_Types.Root_Controlled with null record;

    procedure Initialise (Object : in out Controlled);
    procedure Duplicate (Object : in out Controlled) is <>;
    procedure Finalize (Object : in out Controlled) is <>;
end Finalization;
```

The purpose of the *Duplicate* operation is to fix up any pointers or counts after a bit–wise copy has been performed.

4.3. Composition of Program Units

Study Topic S4.3–A(1) – Reducing the Need for Recompilation: Ada 9X recompilation and related rules should be revised so it is easier for implementations to minimise the need for recompilation and for programmers to use program structures that reduce the need for recompilation.

Discussion: One cause of excessive recompilation is the inability to decompose a large package specification because the of the need to share private declarations. In Ada 9X, the concept of child library units have been added to achieve this.

A package, *Parent*, can have a child unit (called for example *Parent.Child*). The key property of a child unit is that is can see the private declarations of its parent, thus allowing a large specification to be decomposed, thereby reducing recompilation when parts of the original specification change.

A package, can also have a private child, which can be accessed from the parent package body, any unit descended from the parent but no other unit – this allows a large body to be decomposed, further reducing the need for recompilation.

The fact that a generic package can have (generic) children offers a corresponding benefit for large generic package specifications and/or bodies.

A further benefit of the child library unit facility is that it helps to overcome the restriction that all library units must have distinct names.

Tagged types also contribute (q.v.).

Study Topic S4.3–B(1) – Programming by Specialisation/Extension: Ada 9X shall make it possible to define new declared entities whose properties are adapted from those of existing entities by addition or modification of properties or operations in such a way that: the original entity's definition and implementation are not modified; and the new entity (or instances thereof) can be used anywhere the original one could be, in exactly the same way.

Discussion: Tagged types have been added to achieve this. A record type can be designated as tagged:

> **type** *T1* **is tagged record ... end record;**

Such a type can be extended with extra components:

> **type** *T2* **is new** *T1* **with record ... end record;**

The primitive operations of a tagged type are (just as for derived types), those declared in the same package specification. When a type is derived, it can inherit the primitive operations of its parent or can override some of them and create more primitive types.

Run–time dispatching only occurs when an object of type $T'Class$ is involved. $T'Class$ is the type whose values are the union of all the descendent types of T, ie all those types (directly or indirectly) derived from T. An object of a type descended from T can be (implicitly or explicitly) converted to type $T'Class$, so given:

> **package** *P* **is**
>   **type** *T1* **is tagged record ... end record;**
>   **procedure** *Proc (Param : T1);*
> **end** *P;*

```
package Q is
    type T5 is new T1 with record ... end record;
    procedure Proc (Param : T5);
end P;
```

then in the following procedure, if *Param* is of type *P.T1*, then the procedure *P.Proc* will be called, and if *Param* is of type *Q.T5*, then procedure *Q.Proc* will be called.

```
procedure PP (Param : P.T1'Class) is
begin
    P.Proc (Param);
end PP;
```

Study Topic S4.3–C(1) – Enhanced Library Support: Ada 9X shall make it easier for implementations to provide improved library management support and when possible, shall improve the uniformity with which such support is provided.

Discussion: No improved library management support has been included.

4.4. Generics

Study Topic S4.4–A(1) – Generic Formal Parameters: Ada 9X should enhance generics to liberalise the uses of generic formal parameters within the template, and/or to allow more kinds of formal parameters, in the interest of improving the language's abstraction facilities.

Discussion: In Ada 9X, a generic package can have formal package parameters, so if *GP* and *Gen_Pack* are generic packages, such as:

```
generic
    type T is private;
package GP is ...

generic
    type T is private;
    with package GPI is new GP (T);
package Gen_Pack is ...
```

then the following are legal:

```
package GP_Int is new GP (Integer);

package Gen_Pack_Int is new Gen_Pack (Integer, GP_Int);
```

This facility is particularly useful for building abstractions on top of abstractions, for example, building a Complex Elementary Functions package on top of a Complex Types package.

In Ada 9X, a generic package can have also have formal derived type parameters, so if *GP* and *Gen_Pack* are generic packages, such as:

```
generic
    type T1 is new T;
package GP is ...
```

then the following are legal:

```
package GP_T is new Gen_Pack (T);

type New_T is new T;
package GP_New_T is new GP (New_T);
```

Requirement R4.4–B(1) – Dependence on Instantiation of Bodies: A user must have the ability to compile a generic instantiation before compiling the corresponding generic body. In those cases where a body is compiled before the instantiation, the use must have the ability to ensure the unit containing the instantiation is not dependent on the generic body.

Discussion: Such a dependence is now illegal.

Study Topic S4.4–B(2) – Tighten the Contract Model: Ada 9X should ensure that compatibility of a generic instantiation with the corresponding generic body is based solely on the compatibility of each with the generic specification. That is, there should be no cases where the legality of an instantiation depends on how a generic formal is used within the generic body.

Discussion: Cases where the legality of an instantiation depended on the body have been removed, for example in Ada 9X, a distinction is made between definite[1] and indefinite formal subtypes. If the formal is definite, the actual must also be definite; if the formal is indefinite, no objects of the subtype can be declared in the generic body.

Requirement R4.4–C(1) – Generic Code Sharing: Ada 9X shall provide a mechanism (for example a pragma) requesting the sharing or replication of generic code templates. An implementation may place restrictions on the kinds of generic units for which sharing will be permitted.

Discussion: No changes have been made to satisfy this requirement.

4.5. Exceptions

Requirement R4.5–A(1) – Accessing an exception name: The simple name of the most recently raised exception shall be available as a string in an exception handler. If additional information (such as the name of the unit where the exception was raised) can be made available at little implementation cost, this would also be helpful.

Discussion: Language–defined subprograms have been defined in package *System.Exceptions* to achieve this, together with the exception choice parameter, for example:

```
exception
   when X : others =>
      Put (System.Exceptions.Exception_Name (X));
end;
```

4.6. Input/Output

Requirement R4.6–A(1) – Interactive *Text_Io*: Ada 9X shall improve the ability of Ada programs to communicate with users via interactive devices. Among the capabilities to be considered are: the ability to output text and receive text input on the same line; ensuring that column, line and page numbers reflect use of the same device for input and

---

[1]A subtype is definite if it is either a constrained subtype, or an unconstrained subtype with defaults for all discriminants.

for output; and the ability to continue execution other tasks while one task is waiting for input.

Discussion: No changes have been included to satisfy this requirement.

Requirement R4.6–B(1) – Additional Input/Output Functions: Ada 9X shall augment Ada's input/output functionality in ways that make the capabilities easier to use.

Discussion: Four functions are identified in the Requirements Document for consideration:

(a) *the ability to check whether a file exists (without having to open it)*: no changes have been included to satisfy this requirement.

(b) *a standard way to open a file for appending data to it*: the subtype *File_Mode* has an extra literal, *Append_File*, for specifying this.

(c) *the ability to determine the maximum line length and page length for a given text file*: no changes have been included to satisfy this requirement.

(d) *the ability to read or write different types of data to the same external sequential file*: a general stream–oriented I/O package is provided to support heterogeneous I/O.

5.   Real–Time Requirements

5.1.   Time

Requirement R5.1–A(1) – Elapsed Time Measurement: Ada 9X constructs that deal with time shall support two abstractions of time – monotonically increasing elapsed time and the time of day. The time of day abstraction shall be compatible with the Ada 83 package *Calendar* and may be maintained with different precision from that of elapsed time.

Discussion: The concept of monotonic time has been introduced via package *System.Real_Time*, defined in the Real–Time Systems Annex.

Requirement R5.1–B(1) – Precise Periodic Execution: Ada 9X shall provide a standard way to control the periodic execution of a sequence of statements with respect to elapsed time and the time of day. The method provided shall allow the period to be changed during the execution of a program and shall ensure that the statements are scheduled for execution at precisely the specified time.

Discussion: This can be achieved via the *delay–until* construct, for example:

```
declare
    Increment : System.Real_Time.Fine_Duration := ...;
    Next_Time : System.Real_Time.Time := System.Real_Time.Clock
begin
    loop
        Next_Time := Next_Time + Increment;
        delay until Next_Time;
        [sequence_of_statements]
    end loop;
end;
```

A similar effect can be achieved using package *Calendar*:

```
declare
    Increment : Calendar.Duration := ...;
    Next_Time : Calendar.Time := Calendar.Clock
begin
    loop
        Next_Time := Next_Time + Increment;
        delay until Next_Time;
        [sequence_of_statements]
    end loop;
end;
```

Requirement R5.1–C(1) – Detection of Missed Deadlines: Ada 9X shall facilitate the detection of missed deadlines and the ability to initiate an appropriate response.

Discussion: This can be achieved via the asynchronous transfer of control facility:

```
select
    delay 1.0;
    [sequence–of_statements]
then abort
    [abortable_sequence_of_statements]
end select;
```

The delay statement and the abortable sequence of statements are executed in parallel. If the delay expires before the abortable sequence of statements completes, the latter is aborted. If the abortable sequence of statements completes before the delay expires, the delay is cancelled.

5.2. Task Scheduling

Requirement R5.2–A(1) – Alternative Scheduling Algorithms: Ada 9X shall allow real–time programmers to determine the scheduling policy and algorithm to be used for a particular program.

Discussion: The Real–Time Systems Annex defines pragmas *Task_Dispatching_Policy* and *Queueing_Policy* with an extensible set of argument values – other scheduling algorithms can added by an implementation by the use of pragmas.

Requirement R5.2–A(2) – Common Real–Time Paradigms: Ada 9X shall ensure that common real–time paradigms can be implemented with predictably efficient performance. Among the paradigms to be considered are: controlling access to data shared among different tasks, resetting task priorities in response to a mode change, critical regions, and asynchronous communication.

Discussion: The Protected Type construct (see [5]) has been added to enable various common paradigms to be readily captured.

5.3. *Asynchronous Control of Execution*

Requirement R5.3–A(1) – Asynchronous Transfer of Control: Ada 9X shall allow the execution of a sequence of statements to be abandoned in order to execute a different sequence within the same task. The event causing this transfer might be, for example, an external interrupt from a timer or a call from another task. It shall be possible to abandon the execution quickly, even if execution is suspended at an entry call or accept statement. In balancing the need for immediate response with the need for safe and predictable execution (eg the ability to release resources held by the abandoned code), it shall be possible to identify certain sections of code in which a request for asynchronous transfer of control will be honoured.

Discussion: Such a facility has been added.

```
select
    [entry_call_statement]
    [sequence-of_statements]
then abort
    [abortable_sequence_of_statements]
end select;
```

The entry call statement and the abortable sequence of statements are executed in parallel. If the entry call is accepted before the abortable sequence of statements completes, the latter is aborted. If the abortable sequence of statements completes before the entry call is accepted, it is cancelled.

5.4. *Asynchronous Communication*

Requirement R5.4–A(1) – Non–Blocking Communication: Ada 9X shall support non-blocking, asynchronous communication between tasks in an Ada program. In particular, from the viewpoint of the sending task, the maximum time to execute an asynchronous communication operation shall normally be independent of the state of the receiving task.

Discussion: This can be achieved via the Protected Types facility (see [5]).

Study Topic S5.4–B(1) – Asynchronous Multicast: Ada 9X shall support asynchronous communication from a single sender to multiple receivers as well as the ability of potential receivers to control their eligibility to receive a message.

Discussion: This can be achieved via the Protected Types facility (see [5]).

6.   Requirements for System Programming

6.1.   Unsigned Integer Operations

Requirement R6.1–A(1) – Unsigned Integer Operations: Ada 9X shall provide efficient support for operations on unsigned integer data. In particular, unsigned arithmetic, logical operations, and shifting operations shall be supported.

Discussion: Ada 9X has an explicit unsigned integer type, for example a 16–bit unsigned integer type can be declared thus:

> **type** *Unsigned* **is mod** *2**16;*

6.2.   Data Interoperability

Requirement R6.2–A(1) – Data Interoperability: Ada 9X shall provide a means to specify the exact representation of data in memory and on external files so that interoperability with other systems can be facilitated.

Discussion: Stream Input–Output has been added to support interoperability.

6.3.   Interrupts

Requirement R6.3–A(1) – Interrupt Servicing: Ada 9X shall ensure that an interrupt can be serviced with minimal (and predictable) run–time overhead. Ada 9X shall allow interrupts to be processed at an appropriate priority.

Discussion: This can be achieved by associating a pragma *Attach_Handler* (defined in the Systems Programming Annex) with a protected parameterless procedure and supplying a pragma *Interrupt_Priority* (defined in the Real–Time Systems Annex), for example:

```
protected Object is
    entry Read (D : out Data);
    pragma Interrupt_Priority (15);
private
    procedure Handle;
    pragma Attach_Handler (Handler, Interrupt_Id);
    Value : Data;
    Value_Available : Boolean := False;
end Object;
```

Requirement R6.3–A(2) – Interrupt Binding: Ada 9X shall allow the association between an interrupt and its interrupt–handling code to be modified during program execution.

Discussion: Dynamic association between an interrupt and a handler can be achieved by associating a pragma *Interrupt_Handler* with a protected parameterless procedure and using the facilities of package *Interrupt_Management* (both defined in the Systems Programming Annex), for example:

```
protected Object_2 is
    entry Read (D : out Data);
    procedure Attach (Interrupt : System.Interrupt.Interrupt_Id);
private
    procedure Handle;
    pragma Interrupt_Handler (Handler);
    Value : Data;
    Value_Available : Boolean := False;
end Object_2;
```

with the body of procedure *Attach*, taking the form:

```
procedure Attach (Interrupt : System.Interrupts.Interrupt_Id) is
begin
    System.Interrupts.Attach_Handler (New_Handler => Handler'Access;
                                      Interrupt => Interrupt);
end Attach;
```

6.4. Dynamic References to Global Objects

Requirement R6.4–A(1) – Access Values Designating Global Objects: Ada 9X shall allow the use of access values that designate objects declared in library packages. Operations using such access values shall maintain the reliability and safety of Ada 83 access types.

Discussion: This can be achieved via general access (or "access–to–data") types , that can designate both static and dynamic objects. A general access type (indicated by one of the reserved words **all** and **constant**) takes the form:

```
type T_Ptr is access all T;

type Constant_T_Ptr is access constant T;
```

They enable objects of that type to designate both heap and stack objects, the latter only if the designated object is declared to be **aliased** (which allows the *'Access* attribute to be applied). If the keyword **constant** is used, then the value of the designated object cannot be changed via access objects of that type – it may of course change its value either directly or via non–constant access objects.
    The following is then possible:

```
T_Object : aliased T;

Ptr : T_Ptr := T_Object'Access;

Constant_Ptr : Constant_T_Ptr := T_Object'Access;

Ptr.all := 10;

Ptr := new T;
```

Study Topic S6.4–B(1) – Low–Level Pointer Operations: Ada 9X shall provide low-level mechanisms for manipulating pointers.

Discussion: This capability has not been provided.

7.   Requirements for Parallel Processing

7.1.   Shared Memory

Requirement R7.1–A(1) – Control of Shared Memory: Ada 9X must permit an Ada programmer to control access to shared memory and to make full use of shared memory.

Discussion: Four pragmas have been defined in the Systems programming Annex to achieve this: *Atomic*, *Volatile*, *Atomic_Components* and *Volatile_Components*.

These pragmas can be applied to a type or to an object. For an atomic object (or component), all reads and writes of the object as a whole are indivisible. For a volatile object, all reads and writes of the object as a whole are performed directly to memory.

7.2.   Massively Parallel Architectures

Study Topic S7.2–A(1) – Managing Large Numbers of Tasks: Ada 9X must provide for the efficient creation, initialisation, execution and termination of large numbers of tasks.

Discussion: Task discriminants enable a task to have an initial value, so removing the need for sequentialising the initialisation by calling an initialising entry. Note that array iterators, which enabled an index to be passed to an array component were removed from the language due to unjustifiable negative impact.

7.3.   Vector Architectures

Study Topic S7.3–A(1) – Statement Level Parallelism: Ada 9X should accommodate compiler techniques for efficient mapping sequences of Ada statements, including particularly appropriate loops, onto vector architectures.

Discussion: No change has been made to achieve this.

7.4.   Configuration of Parallel Programs

Study Topic S7.4–A(1) – Configuration of Parallel Programs: Ada 9X compilation systems should permit the programmer to optionally control the assignment of Ada tasks to separate processing elements in a multi–processor system.

Discussion: No change has been made to achieve this.

8. Requirements for Distributed Processing

8.1. Distribution of Ada Applications

Requirement R8.1–A(1) – Facilitating Software Distribution: Ada 9X shall facilitate the distribution of Ada code across a homogeneous distributed architecture.

Discussion: The concept of a partition helps in the distribution of a program across a set of homogeneous processors. Three examples of enhancements to facilitate distribution were given:

(a) *the specification of the exact semantics (behaviour and timing, including failure semantics) of timed and conditional entry calls, potentially remote subprograms calls and exception propagation*: the semantics are defined in the Distributed Systems Annex.

(b) *the specification of semantics to deal with hardware failure and recovery*: other than specify that exception Communication_Error be raised if a remote call cannot be completed due to difficulties in communicating with the called partition, this is not addressed.

(c) *treatment of the existence of independent clocks with possibly different timing precisions*: this is not addressed.

8.2. Dynamic Reconfiguration of Distributed System

Requirement R8.2–A(1) – Dynamic Reconfiguration: Ada 9X shall allow for the possibility of dynamic reconfiguration of a distributed application. It shall, be possible to replace or modify individual components of a distributed application without recompiling or restarting the entire application.

Discussion: The concepts of partition and pre–elaboration help this, but the requirement is not directly addressed.

9. Requirements for Safety–Critical and Trusted Applications

9.1. Predictability of Execution

Study Topic S9.1–A(1) – Determining Implementation–Dependent Choices: Wherever Ada 9X *explicitly* allows implementation–defined choices that affect program behaviour, implementors shall be required either to document the choice that has been made (or the situations that control what choice is made) or Ada 9X shall provide a mechanism for controlling the choice.

Discussion: The Safety and Security Annex states that "The implementation shall document the range of effects for each situation that the language rules identify as either a bounded error or as having an unspecified effect". It advises that "among the situations that should be documented are the conventions chosen for parameter passing, the methods used for the management of run–time storage, and the method used to evaluate numeric expressions if this involves extended range or extra precision".

Requirement R9.1–A(2) – Ensuring Canonical Application of Operations: Ada 9X shall provide a mechanism, applicable to a region of program text, for restricting any freedom otherwise allowed to reorder, replace or remove actions involving predefined operations.

Discussion: This requirement is partially satisfied by pragma *Inspection_Point*, defined in the Safety and Security Annex, which identifies a set of named objects, whose values are to be available during execution at the point of the pragma. No dead–code elimination is possible on the variable.

9.2. Certifiability

Requirement R9.2–A(1) – Generating Easily Checked Code: Ada 9X shall provide a mechanism for advising a compiler that code should be generated in a style that allows it to be checked against the source text with reasonable effort.

Discussion: Pragma *Reviewable*, defined in the Safety and Security Annex, requires an implementation to provide certain information both in a human–readable form and in a format suitable for processing by automated tools. The information includes identifying compiler–generated run–time checks, possibly uninitialised variables and providing an object code listing.

9.3. Enforcement of Safety–Critical Programming Practices

Requirement R9.3–A(1) – Allow Additional Compile–Time Restrictions: Ada 9X shall allow a mode in which a compiler enforces adherence to coding practices beyond those imposed by the rules of the language.

Discussion: Pragma *Restrictions* is defined in Section 13 of the Reference Manual. The Safety and Security Annex defines a set of arguments to the pragma, such as *No_Protected_Types, No_Allocators, No_Floating_Point*.

10.   Requirements for Information Systems

10.1. Predictability of Execution

Requirement R10.1–A(1) – Decimal–Based Types: Ada 9X shall support fixed point types whose value of *small* is a power of ten. Such types shall have at least 18 decimal digits of precision. It shall be possible to ensure that intermediate results for expressions of such types are not computed or stored with extra precision, and that rounding is under programmer control.

Discussion: Ada 9X includes special syntax to declare decimal types. The Information Systems Annex defines a specifiable attribute (*Machine_Radix*) that requires an implementation to support a radix of 10, for example:

> **type** *Money* **is delta** *0.01* **digits** *15;*
> **for** *Money'Machine_Radix* **use** *10;*

Study Topic S10.2–A(2) – Specification of Decimal Representation: Ada 9X information system implementations shall provide a mechanism for specifying decimal representations for decimal–based fixed point types.

Discussion: Ada 9X advises implementations that support a radix of 10 to use a packed decimal representation.

10.2. Compatibility with Other Character Sets

Study Topic S10.2–A(1) – Alternate Character Set Support: Ada 9X information-system implementations shall provide for the extension of the set of graphic symbols to obtain input/output facilities and *Image* attributes for alternate character sets (specifically for *Ebcdic*) comparable in both functionality and performance with the features provided for the built–in character set.

Discussion: A package to support *Latin–1* is defined in the Predefined Language Environment (Annex C). Packages to support *EBCDIC* and *PC* were removed during the Mapping Phase.

10.3. Interfacing with Data Base Systems

Study Topic S10.3–A(1) – Interfacing with Data Base Systems: It should be relatively easy to write Ada 9X programs that interface smoothly with DBMSs.

Discussion: Data interoperability formats are supported.

10.4. Common Functions

Study Topic S10.4–A(1) – Varying–Length String Package: Ada 9X shall provide a standard varying–length string package.

Discussion: Three packages are defined in the Predefined Language Environment (Annex C): *Strings.Fixed* for fixed–length strings, *Strings.Bounded* for strings whose upper bound can vary from zero to a maximum size established at instantiation time, and *Strings.Unbounded* whose upper bound can vary from zero to *Natural'Last*.

Study Topic S10.4–A(2) – String Manipulation Functions: Ada 9X shall provide a standard package of general string manipulation functions such as a function for finding a pattern in a string, a conversion function, and functions for creating formatted data in the style of "picture" formats as specified in languages such as *COBOL* and *PL/1*.

Discussion: The three packages *Strings.Fixed*, *Strings.Bounded* and *Strings.Unbounded* define operations for finding a pattern in a string and for a conversion function. A package (*Text_Io.Picture_Io*) is defined in the Information Systems Annex for text input and picture–based output of values of a decimal type.

11. Requirements for Scientific and Mathematical Applications

11.1. Floating Point

Requirement R11.1–A(1) – Standard Mathematics Packages: Ada 9X shall provide a standard package of elementary functions such as sine, cosine, square root, logarithm etc. In addition, Ada 9X shall provide a standard interface to subprograms that are useful in developing portable implementations of mathematical functions.

Discussion: A package (*Numerics.Generic_Elementary_Functions*) is defined in the Predefined Language Environment (Annex C), almost identical to that standardised for Ada 83 to define elementary functions such as sine, cosine, square root, logarithm, etc.

The Numerics Annex defines a set of primitive function attributes, such as *Exponent, Fraction, Compose, Floor, Ceiling*, etc.

Study Topic S11.1–B(1) – Floating Point Facilities: Ada 9X shall require that the results of following point operations shall be predictable from the documentation provide for any given implementation. Ada 9X shall also allow implementations to fully support the IEEE floating point standard.

Discussion: The floating point model has been remove from the core language to the Numerics and modified to address these requirements.

11.2. Representation of Arrays

Study Topic S11.2–A(1) – Array Representation: Ada 9X shall allow programmers to determine whether arrays are organised in row–major or column–major order.

Discussion: The Language Interface packages Annex specifies that arrays are organised in the Fortran manner if pragma Convention (Fortran) applies, for example:

```
type Fortran_Matrix is array (Integer range <>, Integer range <>) of Double_Precision;
pragma Convention (Fortran, Fortran_Matrix);
```

References

[1] ANSI/MIL–STD 1815A, Reference Manual for the Ada Programming Language, January 1983.
[2] Ada 9X Project Report, Ada 9X Requirements Document, Department of Defense, December 1990.
[3] Ada 9X Project Report, Ada 9X Requirements Rationale, Department of Defense, May 1991.
[4] Ada 9X Reference Manual, Draft Version 3.0, Intermetrics, 29 June 1993.
[5] Ada 9X Project Report, Introducing Ada 9X, Department of Defense, February 1993.

Ada: Towards Maturity
Ed. L. Collingbourne
IOS Press 1993

Object-Oriented Programming and Ada 9X: What can we learn from C++?

John English
Department of Computing
University of Brighton, Lewes Road, Brighton BN2 4GJ, England
E-mail: je@unix.brighton.ac.uk

Abstract. One of the most important new features proposed for Ada 9X is the inclusion of support for object-oriented programming. C++ is a descendant of C which supports object-oriented programming and which is now established as one of the major object-oriented languages. Like Ada 9X, C++ is a development of an existing procedural language which imposes the need for it to provide backward compatibility. Unlike Ada 9X, C++ has been available now for a number of years and a great deal of experience of its usefulness in practice has been acquired. This paper presents a comparison of the features of Ada 9X and C++ which are intended to support object-oriented programming. It examines the object-oriented features of C++ and considers whether the features proposed for Ada 9X can provide the expressive power of C++ while at the same time avoiding the complexities arising from C++'s incremental evolution. In addition, it describes some of the problems encountered with C++ in practice and explains how the practical lessons learnt from C++ might be applied to the future use of Ada 9X.

1. Introduction.

Object-oriented programming has become an extremely important programming paradigm in recent years which promises improvements in productivity, maintainability and code reusability. Developed originally from the class construct of Simula 67 [1], the concepts involved were developed further in Smalltalk [2] which is arguably the first truly object-oriented language. More recently, languages like Objective-C [3] and C++ [4,5] have added object-oriented features to existing languages. C++ has become a particularly important language by virtue of its widespread availability and the fact that it is based on C. One of the major changes to be introduced in Ada 9X [6,7] is the incorporation of features to supported the object-oriented programming paradigm. This paper describes the object-oriented features of C++ and compares them to the facilities proposed for Ada 9X.

C++ has been widely used for several years now, and has evolved considerably in the process. It is a rich and complex language — rich in features which have been added as experience with using the language showed them to be necessary or desirable, and complex due to the interaction of these features. Unlike C++, Ada 9X has been carefully planned as a whole rather than evolving incrementally, but this means that there is as yet no practical experience of using the language to solve real problems. Various practical difficulties have been identified in C++ as a result of using the language to solve real problems, and this paper discusses these difficulties and considers to what extent they might apply to Ada 9X.

2. Comparing C++ with Ada 9X.

2.1. *Object-oriented programming.*

Object-oriented programming is a natural extension of the use of abstract data types. Object-oriented programs are composed of a number of interacting *objects* each of which belongs to a particular *class*. A class is essentially an abstract data type. However, it is possible to define a new *derived* class as an extension of an existing class which *inherits* all the characteristics of the *base class* from which it is derived. Derived classes can in turn act as the base class for further derivation, resulting in a hierarchy of related classes. (Note that this terminology is that used in C++; there is as yet no completely standardised terminology for object-oriented programming.)

An object of a derived class will contain the data members inherited from its base class, and can define extra data members in addition to these. All the operations which apply to an object of the base class can also be applied to the derived class; the derived class can define additional primitive operations and can also redefine inherited operations by overloading. This technique is sometimes referred to as *programming by extension.*

Since the derived class is an extension of the base class, derived class objects can be used in any context where a base class object is required. One of the major benefits of object-oriented programming is *polymorphism*, where the actual type of an object is used at run-time to select the correct version of an operation for that object. If a base class declares a primitive operation P, classes derived from it can overload P to provide appropriate behaviour for their particular circumstances. If P is then applied to each of a heterogenous collection of objects belonging to these derived classes, the version of P executed in each case will depend on the actual type of object to which it was being applied with the correct version being selected dynamically at run-time. Further derived classes can be declared at a later date which also overload P in a new way, and the code to process the collection will still work correctly with these new derived classes without any changes (not even recompilation) being necessary.

Whereas Smalltalk is a "pure" object-oriented language (where everything ultimately derives from the class Object), C++ and Ada 9X are both developments of conventional procedural languages into object-oriented languages, and as such have a requirement for the greatest possible degree of backward compatibility to their ancestors C and Ada 83. Both languages are statically typed (i.e. object types are resolved at compile-time) whereas Smalltalk is dynamically typed, with all type resolution being done at run-time. Smalltalk is therefore able to exploit the object-oriented paradigm in a full-blooded fashion impossible in either C++ or Ada 9X; for example, False and True in Smalltalk are not values, they are classes derived from Boolean which overload the methods *ifTrue:* and *ifFalse:* to either execute or ignore the supplied argument as appropriate.

2.2. *Classes in C++.*

C++ was developed by Bjarne Stroustrup in the late 1970s as an extension of C [8]. Originally called "C with Classes", it borrowed from Simula's class construct to add class declarations to C. It has since become widely available and extremely popular. Experience with using the language has resulted in a series of incremental language revisions, with version 3.0 being the most recent version. C++ is currently undergoing standardisation, with an ANSI standard expected in the near future.

C++ has used an extension of *struct* (record) types to provide its object-oriented features; a C++ class declaration declares a data type which specifies both the data members of an object belonging to that class and a set of *member functions* which can be applied to objects of that type. C has no equivalent to the package construct of Ada, so C++ uses class declarations to provide the encapsulation and access control facilities which are provided by packages in Ada. The member functions of a C++ class are declared within the class declaration but are defined separately, in a similar way to the separation of package specifications and bodies in Ada.

Like C++, Ada 9X extends the notion of record types to provide type extensibility with the introduction of *tagged types*, but unlike C++ these play no part in controlling encapsulation or visibility. This is the root cause of many of the differences in approach to object-oriented programming in the two languages.

Visibility in C++ classes is provided by specifying class members as being *public, private* or *protected*, where only the public members of a class can be accessed by clients of the class. Private members can only be accessed by the class member functions (or "friends" of the class, as described below), while protected members are also accessible to any derived classes.

Member selection is accomplished using the same "dot" notation as for Ada records, which is extended to include member functions. A member function is thus always called with reference to a specific "current object" as an implicit extra parameter, and within the definition of the member function unqualified references to class members implicitly refer to the members of the current object. This is essentially the same approach as is taken in Smalltalk. The special pointer *this* yields a pointer to the current object, corresponding to *self* in Smalltalk.

Ada 9X does not use this "distinguished receiver" approach; C++ member functions would be written in Ada 9X as normal subprograms with all parameters specified explicitly. This is another consequence of separating encapsulation issues from extensibility issues.

Figure 1 gives an outline of a C++ class to represent a simple bank account which will be used to illustrate many of the features discussed in this section, and shows the declaration of a BankAccount object and a call to a member function. It is intended as a base class from which specific types of bank accounts (current accounts, savings accounts and so on) can be derived. Figure 2 shows the outline of an equivalent Ada 9X package.

2.3. Virtual functions.

Since derived classes in C++ can be used wherever an object of the base class is expected, a function expecting a parameter which refers to a base class object can always be called with a reference to a derived class object instead. If the function calls a member function of the class, the compiler will normally resolve this into a call of the base class member function since the apparent type of the parameter is that of the base class. If the member function has been overloaded in the derived class this will not produce the desired behaviour. What is required here is a polymorphic mechanism which uses the actual type of the parameter to identify the correct version of the member function dynamically at run-time.

Polymorphism in C++ classes is accomplished by declaring polymorphic functions to be *virtual* in the base class. Functions declared to be virtual will be subject to polymorphic run-time dispatching; other (non-virtual) functions will be bound at compile time based on the apparent type of the objects for which the operation is being invoked. Thus if the member

```
class BankAccount
{
  public:
    BankAccount            (Name_t who);     // open account
    virtual ~BankAccount   ();               // close account
    virtual void withdraw  (Money_t amount); // withdraw money
    virtual void deposit   (Money_t amount); // deposit money
    Money_t      balance   ();               // query balance
    ...
  private:
    Name_t    name;        // account holder's name
    Number_t  number;      // account number
    Money_t   amount;      // current balance
    ...
};

BankAccount john ("John English");    // declare a BankAccount object
john.withdraw (100.00);               // withdraw some money
```

Figure 1: Outline BankAccount class declaration and usage in C++.

```
package BANK_ACCOUNT_PKG is
   type BANK_ACCOUNT is tagged limited private;
   procedure OPEN   (ACCT: in out BANK_ACCOUNT;
                     NAME: in NAME_TYPE);          -- open account
   procedure CLOSE (ACCT: in out BANK_ACCOUNT);   -- close account
   procedure WITHDRAW (ACCT: in out BANK_ACCOUNT;
                     AMOUNT: in out MONEY);        -- withdraw money
   procedure DEPOSIT   (ACCT: in out BANK_ACCOUNT;
                     AMOUNT: in out MONEY);        -- deposit money
   function  BALANCE   (ACCT: BANK_ACCOUNT) return MONEY;
                                                   -- query balance
   ...
private
   type BANK_ACCOUNT is tagged record
      NAME    : NAME_TYPE;
      NUMBER  : NUMBER_TYPE;
      AMOUNT  : MONEY;
   end record;
end BANK_ACCOUNT_PKG;
```

Figure 2: Outline BankAccount package in Ada 9X.

function *withdraw* were applied to a collection of different sorts of bank accounts, the version of *withdraw* appropriate for each account in the collection would be called. The base class definition of *balance* would always be used, however.

Ada 9X uses a different mechanism (*class-wide* operations) to achieve the same effect. The implications of this are explored further in section 3 below.

2.4. Constructors and destructors.

A C++ class can contain special member functions known as *constructors* and *destructors*. Constructors and destructors are named after their class; the constructor for class *BankAccount* is called *BankAccount* and the destructor is called *~BankAccount*. There can be several overloaded constructors but only a single destructor. These functions perform initialisation and finalisation for objects of the class. By using a constructor to initialise objects when they are declared, the risk of forgetting to initialise them before use is eliminated. A constructor is called when an object is declared, and so cannot return a result (since a declaration cannot form part of an expression). Any parameters to the constructor can be used to initialise the object.

The destructor is called automatically whenever an object is destroyed; consequently, destructors cannot return a result or take any parameters. Typical actions which might be performed by destructors include the deallocation of heap space used by objects, unhooking interrupt vectors if interrupt handlers have been installed, deleting a window on a screen in a graphical user interface, or printing a closing statement for a bank account.

Tagged types in Ada 9X do not in general have an equivalent to constructors and destructors, and so procedures *OPEN* and *CLOSE* are provided instead in Figure 2. However, destructors can be provided by inheritance from the limited type CONTROLLED and parameterised constructors can sometimes be modelled using discriminants. These issues are discussed in greater detail in section 4 below.

2.5. Operator overloading.

C++ introduces the ability to overload operators in a similar manner to Ada. In some ways it is a more restrictive facility than in Ada; at least one of the operands of an overloaded operator must belong to a user-defined class type, and the result type of the operator is not considered in overload resolution due to the fact that any expression can be used as a statement and so the result type would not necessarily be determinable when applying the operator.

In other ways C++ is less restrictive than Ada in the range of operators which are considered overloadable. These include the assignment operator, function call brackets, subscript brackets, the comma operator and type conversion operators. While some of these (notably assignment and subscript brackets) can prove extremely useful to overload, they can easily be misused. The ability to define automatic type conversions as operators is particularly dangerous, as they will be invoked invisibly by the compiler for the purposes of overload resolution. The source program will not contain any indication that they have been used, which makes it impossible to determine the points at which they are called. This can lead to serious problems when attempting to debug C++ programs.

In Ada the assignment operator ":=" cannot be overloaded. Assignment is provided as a bitwise copy for non-limited types, but for limited types it is necessary to provide a procedure (typically called ASSIGN) to provide the necessary assignment semantics, which in the author's opinion is both ugly and inconsistent. C++ provides a default assignment operator for all types which performs a memberwise copy; assignment can be prohibited where necessary by declaring a private assignment operator or providing a constant as a class member. Alternatives to memberwise copying can be provided by defining a suitable overloading of "operator=" which provides the desired semantics.

2.6. Other features.

It is sometimes necessary or desirable to allow one class to access the private parts of another class, either for efficiency reasons or because the two classes are closely coupled. Typical examples include multiplication of a matrix by a vector, where for efficiency reasons the multiplication operator needs to access the internal representation of both classes to avoid redundant range checks, or collection classes and their iterators where the iterator class needs to be able to access implementation details of the corresponding collection class in order to navigate through the collection while preventing any other class from building in assumptions about the manner in which the collection is actually implemented. A C++ class can specify that another class or function is a friend, which allows the private data of the class to be accessed from within the class or function so nominated. This is necessary as C++ does not provide any separate package-like construct for encapsulation; Ada 9X achieves the effect of friendship by simple encapsulation of the related declarations within the same package.

In our bank account example, we may wish to keep a list of transactions associated with each account. A *Transaction* class could be declared to represent an individual transaction; by making everything private in *Transaction* and declaring *BankAccount* to be a friend of *Transaction*, we can ensure that only *BankAccount* can manipulate *Transaction*s. Note that friendship is not inherited; other classes derived from *BankAccount* will not be able to access members of *Transaction*.

Friends also play a role in operator overloading; a non-friend overloaded operator which needs access to the private part of an object will need to be a class member, in which case the first parameter to the operator must be an object of that class (the implicit "current object" for which the operator is called). Friendship allows operators which are not class members to access the private part of the class. Since Ada 9X does not use the "distinguished receiver" approach of C++, overloaded operators do not need to have a tagged type as their first parameter. There is therefore no need for a special mechanism to address this situation.

C++ also allows members to be declared *static* (thereby adding yet more meanings to an already heavily-overloaded word) which means for a data member that one only copy of it will be created which will be shared by all instances of the class, and for functions means that they will not access non-static members so that they can be used independently of any particular object. For example, class *BankAccount* could use a static member to record the last account number issued. The need for static members is again related to the lack of a separate encapsulation mechanism in C++; a static member corresponds to a variable declared in an Ada package.

2.7. Templates and exceptions.

Two essential features of Ada used in defining abstract data types are generics and exceptions. Generics allow packages to define structures such as linked lists without reference to the actual types of object that the list will hold, while exceptions allow a package to detect errors while delegating the application-specific error handling to the clients of the package.

C++ provides similar but not identical features. *Templates* are analogous to Ada's generics as well as having some similarity to discriminated types. Function and class declarations can be parameterised using types or values. Unlike generics in Ada, templates do not require explicit instantiation before use. Declarations of templated class objects must supply actual values for the template parameters in a similar manner to supplying constraints for a discriminated type in Ada. Templated functions will be instantiated automatically by the

```
template<class T> class Stack
{
  public:
    void push  (T& data);      // push an item onto the stack
    T    pop   ();             // pop an item off the stack
    int  empty ();             // test if stack is empty
    ...
  private:
    ...
};


Stack<int> intstack;           // a stack of integers
```

Figure 3: Outline of a templated Stack class.

compiler wherever necessary. Figure 3 shows an outline of a templated *Stack* class and the declaration of a stack of integers.

Although templates have been part of the official language definition for some time, it is only fairly recently that compilers have appeared which implement them. Of the three most widely used C++ compilers for the IBM PC (Borland, Microsoft and Zortech) only the Borland compiler currently implements templates.

The C++ exception handling mechanism is now part of the official definition of the language.   It is an essentially similar mechanism to exception handling in Ada, and so it is not described further in this paper.   Unfortunately it has not yet been implemented in most compilers due to problems in maintaining compatibility with existing code in both C and C++, although possible implementation strategies have been proposed by Koenig & Stroustrup [9]. This is a serious handicap to writing reusable code in C++ and will require a lot of existing code to be rewritten when exception handling becomes more widely available, which is expected to be sometime in 1994. In the meantime, interim measures have been proposed (e.g. by Bengtsson [10]) which will allow easy migration to exceptions when they become available, but these are invariably inconvenient and messy substitutes for a vitally important mechanism.

3. Inheritance and polymorphism.

3.1. Inheritance and containment.

Inheritance is an extremely elegant mechanism for promoting code reuse. Without inheritance, variant records are needed to gather related types into a single type declaration; without polymorphism it is usually necessary to use a case statement to distinguish between the variants. Adding a new derivation involves modifying the variant record declaration and all of the case statements associated with it, which is an exceedingly error-prone process. Inheritance allows new data types to be implemented by refining existing types, reducing the need for rewriting and testing. Polymorphism allows new derived types to be incorporated in an existing program without affecting any of the existing code. Figure 4 shows a *CurrentAccount* and an *InterestBearingAccount* derived from *BankAccount*; *CurrentAccount* adds an overdraft limit and overloads *withdraw* to check withdrawals against the limit, while

```
class CurrentAccount : public BankAccount
{
  public:
    CurrentAccount (Name_t who) : BankAccount (who)  { }
    virtual void withdraw (Money_t amount);   // withdraw money
    void setOverdraft     (Money_t limit);    // set overdraft limit
  private:
    ...
};

class InterestBearingAccount : public BankAccount
{
  public:
    InterestBearingAccount (Name_t who) : BankAccount (who)  { }
    void accrueInterest ();                      // accrue interest due
  private:
    ...
};
```

Figure 4: CurrentAccount and InterestBearingAccount classes

InterestBearingAccount adds a member function to accrue interest based on the current balance but does not overload anything else.

Inheritance is often characterised as an "is-a" relationship; deriving a derived type D from a base type B implies that D "is-a" B, in other words that D is a kind of B. In Ada 9X, inheritance will make every primitive operation of a base type primitive operations of any type derived from it. It will also be possible to convert from one type to another. Provided that this gives sensible behaviour, inheritance is entirely appropriate. It would not however be sensible to define a Stack as being derived from a LinkedList, since not all LinkedList operations are appropriate for Stacks (and we would not want to be able to interconvert between the two types). C++ muddies the waters slightly by allowing selective exporting of inherited operations using *private inheritance* (see below). A linked list may be used to implement a stack; in this case, the appropriate solution is to include a LinkedList object as a field in the tagged record for Stack. This is an example of a *containment* relationship rather than an inheritance relationship.

As another example, consider a tagged type which represents a point in a Cartesian plane. This could be used as the basis for a point in 3-D space using either containment or inheritance as shown in Figure 5. Either solution is feasible; a 3D_Point is an extension of a 2D_Point (it has one extra coordinate) and it provides operations which correspond to those provided by 2D_Point. Which solution is best depends on whether you want the types to be interconvertible; converting a 3D_Point to a 2D_Point will effectively project the 3D_Point onto a predetermined plane. The main difference is that primitive operations of 2D_Point will not automatically become primitive operations of 3D_Point if containment is used; instead, 3D_Point must define its own set of primitive operations and use the primitive operations of 2D_Point where appropriate.

```
type 2D_Point is tagged record
   X,Y : Coordinate;
end record;
function Distance (A,B : 2D_Point) return Length is
begin        -- return distance between two points
   return Sqrt (abs (A.X - B.X) ** 2 + abs (A.Y - B.Y) ** 2);
end Distance;


--------- Inheriting 3D_Point from 2D_Point
type 3D_Point is new 2D_Point with record
   Z : Coordinate;
end record;
function Distance (A,B : 3D_Point) return Length is
begin
   return Sqrt (Distance (2D_Point(A), 2D_Point(B)) ** 2 +
              abs (A.Z - B.Z) ** 2);
end Distance;


--------- Creating 3D_Point from 2D_Point by containment
type 3D_Point is record
   XY : 2D_Point;
   Z  : Coordinate;
end record;
function Distance (A,B : 3D_Point) return Length is
begin
   return Sqrt (Distance (A.XY, B.XY) ** 2 + abs (A.Z - B.Z) ** 2);
end Distance;
```

Figure 5: 2D_Point and 3D_Point classes

3.2. Access control.

C++ allows the exporting of members inherited from a base class to be controlled by specifying the derived class as being a public, private or protected derivation of a base class. With private inheritance, all public and protected members of the base class become private members of the derived class. Protected inheritance makes public and protected members of the base class protected members of the derived class, and public inheritance means that all base class members continue to have the same access in the derived class as they had in the base class. Derived classes can also selectively alter the access to individual members inherited from a base class.

   Access control in Ada 9X is essentially the same as in Ada 83. In Ada 83, the private part of a package is only accessible to the corresponding package body. Ada 9X also introduces the notion of *child packages*, which also have access to the private part of their parent packages. This means that the status of the private part of an Ada 9X package is comparable to that of the protected section of a C++ class. Completely private data can only be achieved using opaque types, where an access variable is used to access an object of an incompletely declared type. Figure 6 shows how the private structure of type *BANK_ACCOUNT* can be hidden using an opaque type. This technique has a performance penalty in that the private data must be created

```
package BANK_ACCOUNT_PKG is
   type BANK_ACCOUNT is tagged limited private;
   ...
private
   type BANK_ACCOUNT_DETAILS;        -- incomplete type declaration
   type BANK_ACCOUNT_DETAILS_ACCESS is access BANK_ACCOUNT_DETAILS;
   type BANK_ACCOUNT is tagged record
      DETAILS: BANK_ACCOUNT_DETAILS_ACCESS;
   end record;
end BANK_ACCOUNT_PKG;
```

Figure 6: Using opaque types for private data.

on the heap and later reclaimed. Opaque types can also be used in C++ where they allow the contents of the private part of a class to be altered without the need to recompile all the clients of a class. The C++ class constructor is used to allocate the private data area and the destructor then reclaims it. This is slightly more problematical in Ada 9X where tagged types in general do not have constructors and destructors.

Inheritance in Ada 9X is equivalent to public inheritance in C++; there is no direct equivalent to private and protected inheritance. However, inheritance in C++ is in practice nearly always public (although strangely enough the default is private); private inheritance is generally used to inherit implementations rather than interface, as described in the preceding section, where the full range of operations for the implementation type are inappropriate for the derived type. As noted in the preceding section, this is in general more sensibly done using containment rather than inheritance. It is therefore unlikely that Ada 9X loses any expressive power by providing public inheritance only.

3.3. Virtual functions.

Virtual functions in C++ can prove particularly deceptive. If a function is declared virtual in a base class, any function with the same signature (identical parameter types) is automatically virtual in all classes derived from the base class. The use of the *virtual* keyword is however optional in the derived classes. A common recommendation is to use the *virtual* keyword in the derived classes also; if this is not done, it becomes difficult to distinguish virtual and non-virtual functions. Functions with the same name but a different signature are not automatically virtual; the use of the *virtual* keyword for a previously overloaded name in a derived class may disguise the fact that the derived class is introducing an additional virtual function.

The decision as to which functions should be virtual must be made when the class is designed. Later changes will result in the need not just for recompilation but retesting, as existing calls to a base class function might now end up calling the virtual function in the derived class instead. For example, the *InterestBearingAccount* class derived from *BankAccount* might wish to overload the member function *balance* so that it calculates any interest due whenever the balance is checked in order to avoid running a separate job to pay interest at regular intervals. This would not work properly without changing the declaration of *BankAccount*, since *balance* was not declared as a virtual function. One approach is to make all functions virtual unless there is a very good reason not to, but this can introduce unnecessary inefficiency; virtual function calls involve an extra level of indirection and they cannot in general be expanded inline, thus imposing the overhead of a function entry and exit which might otherwise be avoided.

Ada 9X manages to avoid these problems fairly neatly. Virtual functions have no direct counterpart in Ada 9X; instead, all primitive operations of tagged types (those declared in the same declaration section as the tagged type) are inherited automatically with references to the base type being transformed into corresponding references to the derived type and can be overloaded in the declaration section for the derived type. *Dispatching operations* fulfil the same role as virtual functions in C++. These are calls to primitive operations of a tagged type *T* using a parameter of type *T'CLASS*, which is the set of all types derived from *T*. Primitive operations of *T* and its derivations are selected by using the actual parameter type at run-time to identify the corresponding primitive operation.

In a sense all primitive operations of a tagged type are "virtual" in the C++ sense, as they can all be involved in run-time dispatching. The primitive operations themselves are not responsible for run-time dispatching; dispatching operations are identified at the point of call by the presence of a class-wide parameter. This separation of concerns means that new dispatching operations can be added at any time without affecting existing code. It is also evident by inspection in which situations dispatching occurs.

3.4. Inherited operations.

A derived class in C++ automatically inherits all the data and member functions which apply to the base class, with the exception of the constructors, the assignment operator and the memory allocation operators *new* and *delete*. There are good reasons for not inheriting these operations; if the derived class adds extra data items to the base class, the base class operations will not fulfill the requirements of the derived class. In Ada 9X, operations of this sort (such as functions which return a result of a tagged type) would become *abstract operations* in the derived type. A type containing abstract operations is an abstract type which can be used as a base class for derivation but which cannot have be used to declare instances. The derived type would thus have to redefine these operations before it could be used.

C++ takes a different approach; if the non-inherited operations are not redefined in the derived class, the default operations will be reinstated. In particular, the default assignment operator which performs a member-by-member copy will be used. If a base class has defined an assignment operator to replace the default, reinstating the default operator for its derivations is not a sensible decision and is a source of potential errors in C++.

The mechanism by which operations are inherited from a base class is also slightly different in the two lanaguages. In Ada 9X, when a new type is derived from a tagged type *T* the operations it inherits are obtained by replacing all occurrences of *T* by the name of the new type in the signatures of *T*'s primitive operations. This means that a procedure with two parameters of type *T* is inherited as a procedure with two parameters of the new type. This is somewhat different from the situation in C++, where the parameter types for virtual functions in a derived class must be identical to those in the base class (see Figure 7). This means that a class which provides a virtual function *compare* which takes a reference to a base class object as a parameter must also have a reference to the base class object as its parameter in the derived class so that it ends up as a comparison between a derived class object and a base class object, which is not usually what is required. Proposals have been made to reform this in the final C++ standard to something similar to what Ada 9X does.

```
class Base {
  ...
  virtual int compare (Base& b);     // virtual function
};
Base b;
b.compare (b);                    // base class compared with base class

class Derived : public Base {
  ...
  virtual int compare (Base& b);     // virtual function, same signature
  virtual int compare (Derived& b);  // a new virtual function, not an
};                                   // overload of Base::compare!
Derived d;
d.compare (b);                    // derived class compared with base class
```

Figure 7: Virtual functions with base class parameters.

An interesting parallel between C++ and Ada 9X is that classes are the unit of encapsulation in C++ and it is necessary to choose which functions of a class are polymorphic, while in Ada 9X packages are the unit of encapsulation and it is necessary to choose which types defined in the package are extensible and hence which of the functions in the package are polymorphic.

3.5. Maintenance and reuse issues.

Serious code management problems can arise from the injudicious use of inheritance. Since the derived class only shows the items which differ from the base class, it can be difficult to identify the complete range of behaviour of which a derived class is capable. Locating the definition of a particular member function in a derived class potentially involves inspecting all the classes in its inheritance hierarchy. In such situations, tools such as *class browsers* are an indispensable part of any object-oriented programming environment. Mandatory coding standards are also a good idea; packages which define derived types should contain commentary listing the operations inherited from the base types and indicate which type the operation is inherited from.

Other problems arise from the temptation to devise general-purpose libraries based on Smalltalk-like inheritance hierarchies which use a root class (traditionally called *Object*) from which all other classes are derived. This allows all classes in the hierarchy to share common protocols for behaviour such as persistence, but can lead to severe maintenance and reuse problems in statically-typed languages like C++ and Ada 9X. Each library provider adopting this approach forces users to use their version of *Object*, which may be over-general and inefficient in specific applications. It becomes difficult or impossible to use multiple libraries within a single program. User-defined classes must also be derived from *Object* before they can be used with library features such as collection classes. In Smalltalk, every class is descended from class *Object* and multiple libraries do not exist (the Smalltalk environment itself is the only "library" in Smalltalk), whereas in C++ or Ada 9X there is no global language-defined base class of this sort and hence a need for multiple libraries to satisfy different requirements.

In such a structure the base class quickly becomes bloated. If a class hierarchy is to provide persistence, the basic functions to support it must be present in the root class. These functions will in turn need to rely on other functions and data items, so they must also be present in the base class. The more features the base class tries to provide the larger and more unwieldy it becomes. This is specifically a problem in statically-typed languages like C++ and Ada 9X where all functions which are applicable to a heterogenous collection must be declared in a common base class for the items in the collection.

As an example, the NIHCL class library for C++ [11] is organised in this way. The NIHCL base class *Object* provides facilities for persistent objects and many other features. To do this it includes features such as object type identification, object comparison (although comparing objects which are not of the same type will cause a run-time error to be reported), object printing, persistence, hashing for use by collection classes elsewhere in the hierarchy, and so on. The result is an unwieldy base class which tries to do too many things and loses efficiency in the process. There is a striking parallel here to the way that frequently-used data tends to migrate to a global level in a procedural language so that it can be accessed from anywhere in the program that it is needed; in object-oriented languages, functions tend to migrate into base classes so that they are as widely accessible as possible. It becomes impossible to use a small part of the library (e.g. the *String* class) without using the whole thing; you get type identification and hashing whether you want them or not. Maintenance and readability are also affected because it is necessary to understand most of the features of the library in order to understand a program which uses it.

Multiple inheritance (where a derived class can inherit from a number of base classes) can help achieve some separation of concerns here. Instead of all objects being persistent (which may well be unnecessary), classes which require persistence can be derived from a base class *Persistent* which provides the necessary protocol for achieving persistence, in addition to being derived from any other classes which may be relevant (e.g. class *Printable* if printing is required or class *Collectable* if a hash function must be provided for use by a collection class). Unfortunately, multiple inheritance was added to C++ after NIHCL was developed, so this was not an option for its authors.

3.6. Multiple inheritance.

C++ allows multiple inheritance, whereas Ada 9X has deliberately avoided it in favour of a single inheritance model. Multiple inheritance is a relatively new concept, and as yet there is no single "best" model for it. It is nevertheless an appealing concept which can prove useful in situations such as those described in the previous section. Provided that the base classes are distinct (i.e. they have no common base class themselves) there is little difficulty in implementing multiple inheritance.

When there is a common base class, things can get considerably more difficult. Consider an interest-bearing current account; the simplest way to build one would be to inherit from both *CurrentAccount* and *InterestBearingAccount* so that the functionality of both classes could be combined. Unfortunately in C++ what you get as a result is two separate bank accounts parcelled into one; one will be used as the current account while all the interest is paid into the other. To resolve this problem, C++ overloads the *virtual* keyword once again. The solution is to make *BankAccount* a "virtual public" base class for each of *CurrentAccount* and *InterestBearingAccount*. Only one instance of a virtual base class will be created. The difficulty which then arises is that, in the absence of a crystal ball predicting a future need for multiple inheritance, the declarations of *CurrentAccount* and *InterestBearingAccount* must be altered to accommodate this change when it becomes necessary and all the client code which uses the two classes will then need to be recompiled. Another difficulty in C++ is that the most derived class has the responsibility for calling the virtual base class constructor, which means that all future derivations of *CurrentAccount* and *InterestBearingAccount* will need to know how to construct a *BankAccount* even when multiple inheritance is not being used.

The rationale for omitting multiple inheritance in Ada 9X is described in [6] §4.2.4.4, which lists three possible uses for multiple inheritance: inheriting implementation, *mixin* inheritance and providing multiple views of an object. Inheriting implementation is a bad idea in languages like Ada 9X that do not support selective importing of base class primitives, as mentioned earlier in section 3.1. Mixin inheritance involves the amalgamation of two unrelated classes, a base class and a mixin class. The mixin class provides additional functionality which can be "mixed into" any other suitable base class. As is noted in [6], this can be done in Ada 9X by using a generic package for the mixin class and instantiating with an appropriate base type as its generic parameter. The generic package can then extend the base type as required.

The third situation is where multiple views of a single object are needed. The example given in [6] is a hypertext systems where the type NODE is both a TREE, which enables hypertextual navigation between nodes, and a WINDOW which allows the hypertext to be displayed and interacted with. This scheme involves deriving a new type called STRUCTURE_VIEW from TREE, and deriving a type NODE from WINDOW which includes a STRUCTURE_VIEW member. The embedded STRUCTURE_VIEW member contains a pointer to the NODE which contains it, so that NODE is convertible to type WINDOW, and the embedded STRUCTURE_VIEW member can be manipulated as a TREE and then converted back to a NODE by using the pointer within the STRUCTURE_VIEW. This is a complicated workaround which involves ensuring that the primitives of TREE use access parameters and return class-wide access types as their results so that they can be passed STRUCTURE_VIEW parameters and return pointers to STRUCTURE_VIEWs rather than plain TREEs; TREE must be designed very carefully so that it has the properties required to make the scheme work. With multiple inheritance this could be done simply by using both TREE and WINDOW as base classes without requiring any special properties on their part.

However, none of the examples in [6] address the problem of creating a class such as the interest-bearing current account described above. All the methods described so far would produce an account containing both a current account and an interest-bearing account, which is the problem that virtual base classes are needed to resolve. Although using virtual base classes is a fairly messy business which might mean amending the base classes involved to use virtual inheritance and then recompiling all the code which uses those classes, the alternative in Ada is to derive from *CurrentAccount* and then add the interest-bearing functionality for the derived type. This involves duplicating existing code, assuming the source is available; if it is not then an equivalent algorithm must be devised and tested. Even if the source is available, the duplication of code will lead to maintenance problems as all changes to the original code will need to be replicated in the new class which uses it. The only sensible solution is to abstract the interest-bearing functionality of *InterestBearingAccount* (assuming the source code is available) into a generic package which can then be used as a mixin for both the plain interest-bearing account (a mixin of *BankAccount* with the interest-bearing features) and the interest-bearing current account (a mixin of *CurrentAccount* with the interest-bearing features).

It should be noted that multiple inheritance is in general not a requirement for a successful object-oriented language (for example, Smalltalk does not support it) but it tends to be most heavily used in those languages that support it most easily (e.g. Eiffel [12]). C++ supports it but not in a particularly convenient way, so it is used less in C++ than it might otherwise be. It should also be noted that inheritance itself is not a necessity for object-oriented programming, but its presence makes an object-oriented style a natural way to write programs. Inheritance can be simulated by other means [13] but in languages that do not support it, this style does not come naturally. Multiple inheritance may be similar in that its value is only appreciated where it is usable in a simple and natural manner and that it is only missed if you are already used to it.

4. Creating and destroying objects.

4.1. Constructors and destructors.

The area of initialisation and finalisation of objects is one where Ada 9X and C++ differ most markedly. The differences arise in part from the difference in underlying philosophy in the two languages; C++ is basically expression-oriented and treats declarations as executable statements which can appear at any point within a block, whereas Ada is statement-oriented and rigidly separates declarations from statements. C++ allows classes to have special *constructor* and *destructor* functions which are invoked whenever an object of the corresponding class is created or destroyed. These functions cannot produce any result, and are distinguished by being named after the class they are defined for.

C++ constructors have a number of uses. Apart from being used implicitly to construct objects in declarations, they can also be called explicitly to create temporary objects. Constructors with a single parameter can also act as type conversions from the parameter type to the class type. This can be a problem as the compiler will automatically generate an invisible call to the constructor wherever it thinks such a type conversion is required, with consequent problems when debugging.

C++ classes can also define a special *copy constructor* which will be called whenever an object needs to be copied; for example, when passing an object to a function as an argument or returning an object as the result of a function. Once again, this will be called invisibly by the compiler wherever necessary.

Constructors and destructors allow library developers to ensure that objects are always created and destroyed correctly and can be used to handle some of the implementation details of a class automatically. Unfortunately, there are still situations in C++ where correct behaviour cannot be guaranteed. Global objects in C++ are constructed before entry to the main program and destroyed on exit from the main program. This is similar to the way that package bodies listed in a context clause are elaborated before entering an Ada main program. However, the order of construction of global objects in C++ is linker-dependent if they are declared in separate source files. C++ has no equivalent to the pragma ELABORATE to control the order of elaboration, and must rely on extra-linguistic utilities like linkers which are not under its control. Since linker behaviour is not specified by the language definition, the ordering is in general undefined. Global objects which rely on a particular elaboration sequence are therefore unsafe in C++.

Destruction of objects at program termination can also be a problem. Since C++ uses the same library functions as C, functions such as *exit* and *abort* can know nothing about destructors. The compiler can insert code to ensure that global objects are destroyed as part of the program epilogue code which *exit* executes, but there is insufficient context information to destroy local objects on the stack. *Abort* is a panic exit which does not execute any epilogue code, and so no destructors are called at all. When exceptions become available, local objects will be destroyed in each block that an exception propagates through and the use of functions like *exit* and *abort* will be unnecessary as an exception can be used to unwind the stack and exit the program in an orderly fashion when a fatal error occurs.

4.2. Constructing Ada 9X objects.

Ada 9X does not have constructors or destructors for tagged types. Ada record objects can provide initial values for their components, which can be used to provide the functionality of a C++ parameterless constructor which does nothing more complex than initialise its data members. Constructors with parameters can be simulated to the same extent by providing the tagged type with discriminants which take the place of constructor parameters in C++. Overloaded constructors cannot be simulated directly in Ada 9X. The only general solution is to define constructors and destructors as normal procedures, or for non-limited types to define constructors as functions which can be used as initialisers in declarations.

The difficulty with this approach is that the user must then ensure that the constructor and destructor are explicitly called. The compiler can play no part in ensuring that this is done correctly. For safety, each such type needs a component which indicates whether an object is valid (i.e. it has been constructed but not yet destroyed) which will need checking in each of the primitive operations for that type. This adds yet another burden to the programmer, reduces efficiency due to the need for continual checks, and represents yet another possible source of errors. In addition, exceptions may result in destructor calls being bypassed. There is no way to ensure that a user-supplied destructor procedure will always be called. If heap storage is used (as for example to provide opaque types), this will mean either imposing a burden of responsibility on the programmer or forcing reliance on garbage collection, which is not specifically required by the language and whose presence cannot therefore be guaranteed. Although this is likely to be less than a problem than in C++ (which needs to use heap storage extensively for dynamically-sized arrays) it still poses a problem in Ada 9X. As an illustration, Figure 8 shows a random number generator class in C++ which uses the constructor to determine the range of numbers to be generated and Figure 9 shows some different way of achieving the same effect in Ada 9X.

Automatic initialisation and finalisation can be provided at the cost of making the types involved limited types. Ada 9X provides user-defined initialisation and finalisation for limited types by derivation from the limited type CONTROLLED. Restricting this to limited types ensures that multiple initialisation or finalisation does not occur due to aliasing. Types derived from CONTROLLED inherit the operations INITIALIZE and FINALIZE which are used in much the same way as C++ constructors and destructors. However, INITIALIZE only provides the equivalent of a parameterless constructor in C++.

The lack of multiple inheritance in Ada 9X makes the support for user-defined initialisation and finalisation potentially problematical using this mechanism. If a tagged type *T1* is declared which is not derived from CONTROLLED and at a later date a new tagged type *T2* which requires a destructor is derived from *T1*, *T2* cannot simply be defined as inheriting from both *T1* and CONTROLLED. Instead, the original declaration of *T1* must be modified so that *T1* is derived from CONTROLLED and thus *T2* is also. This will require recompilation of all modules which use the type *T1*. It is in general impossible to predict whether this situation will occur at some future time when a tagged type is being declared. Failing this, the components of *T2* which require finalisation must be aggregated into a separate type derived from

```
class Random
{
  public:
    Random (int low, int high);      // constructor
    int next ();                     // generate next random number
  private:                           // between "low" and "high"
    ...
};

Random dice (1,6);      // declare a random number generator
dice.next ();           // generate a random number between 1 and 6
```

Figure 8: A random number generator class in C++.

```
generic                          -- (a) using generics
   type RANGE_TYPE is range <>;
package RANDOM_PKG is
   type RANDOM is tagged private;
   function NEXT (R: RANDOM) return RANGE_TYPE;
   ...
end RANDOM_PKG;

package RANDOM_PKG is          -- (b) using discriminants
   type RANDOM (LOW, HIGH: INTEGER) is tagged private;
   function NEXT (R: RANDOM) return INTEGER;
   ...
end RANDOM_PKG;

package RANDOM_PKG is          -- (c) using a "constructor" procedure
   type RANDOM is tagged private;
   procedure NEW_RANDOM (LOW, HIGH: in INTEGER);
   function NEXT (R: RANDOM) return INTEGER;
   ...
end RANDOM_PKG;
```

Figure 9: Alternatives to C++ constructors in Ada 9X.

CONTROLLED which can then be used as a component of *T2*. *T2* will still be a limited type, and so may have different behaviour from *T1* (e.g. assignment may be possible for *T1* but will not be for *T2*).

4.3. Controlling object creation.

Constructors and destructors are subject to the same access control mechanisms as other member functions. This means that it is possible to have private or protected constructors and destructors as well as public ones.

Protected constructors can be used to ensure that instances of a base class cannot be created directly but that instances of classes derived from it can be. The same effect can be achieved by

```
class SparseMatrix
{
    friend class SparseItem;
  public:
    SparseItem operator() (int x, int y);
    ...          // subscript operation, produces a SparseItem
};

class SparseItem
{
    friend class SparseMatrix;
  public:
    SparseItem& operator= (float value);   // assignment
    operator float ();                      // type conversion
  private:
    SparseItem (SparseMatrix&, int x, int y);
             // private constructor only accessible to SparseMatrix
};
```

Figure 10: Outline of the SparseMatrix and SparseItem classes

including an abstract operation (what C++ calls a *pure virtual* function). Private constructors only allow friends of the class to create class instances. This is often used to provide *helper* classes. Helper classes are classes which are not directly accessible to users but which play some role in the behaviour of another class. For example, a sparse matrix may allow any of its elements to be selected. Elements which are zero are not stored but can be accessed. If a new value is assigned to a zero element the new element must be stored in the array. The solution here is to have the subscript operation for class *SparseMatrix* return an object of a helper class *SparseItem* which contains a pointer to the array element if it exists or a null pointer if it doesn't and which has a private constructor made accessible only to *SparseMatrix* by means of a *friend* declaration). *SparseItem* can then provide a public assignment operator which can create a new element and add it to the array if a non-zero value is assigned to a zero element. Figure 10 shows an outline of SparseMatrix and SparseItem.

Helper classes cannot be used in this way in Ada 9X. If any operations on a helper type are visible the helper type itself must also be visible, thus allowing users to create objects of the helper type explicitly. The example above would instead require one procedure to extract an individual array element and another procedure to store a new value in a particular element. It would therefore be quite different in appearance and usage from a normal array.

Private destructors prevent objects being created locally. Since the destructor is inaccessible, it cannot be called at the end of the scope in which the declaration occurs and so the compiler will reject the object declaration. The object can be created on the heap using *new* since the compiler does not have to generate a destructor call. The user cannot call *delete* directly since this would invoke the private destructor; instead, a public member function must be defined which can then call *delete* to allow the object to be destroyed. This is occasionally useful, but has no equivalent in Ada 9X.

4.4. Heap management.

C++ programs tend to rely heavily on the heap as this is the only way of creating arrays whose size is not known until run-time. Creating and deleting short-lived heap objects can seriously affect program efficiency, so C++ allows classes to overload the operators *new* and *delete* to allow them to perform memory management in ways more closed suited to their needs. Ada 9X provides a similar ability using *storage pools*.

One of the main problems with overloading *new* in a class is that any further classes derived from it revert to the global definition of *new*. In addition, the global *new* is always used when creating arrays of objects. There is a proposal under consideration by the standards committee which would allow an overloaded version of *new* to be used for creating arrays. It is also necessary to overload *delete* if *new* has been overloaded, but there is nothing in the language to enforce this — it is perfectly possible to overload one without overloading the other. Ada 9X storage pools overcome this problem by defining the ALLOCATE and DEALLOCATE procedures to be abstract subprograms, so that both must be defined in any user-defined storage allocators.

5. Practical problems encountered in C++.

5.1. General problems.

As yet, there can be no practical experience of Ada 9X, but a great deal of experience in using object-oriented programming techniques in C++ has been amassed. Many of the problems encountered in C++ are due to shortcomings of the language in its current form as well as ambiguities in the language specification. The interaction between different features of the language is often unclear, so that (for example) making all possible instantiations of a template class friends of a non-template class may or may not be possible with different compilers according to how the compiler writer has interpreted the language specification.

Some facilities omitted from the language have proved to be necessary in practice. For example, it is sometimes necessary to determine the exact type of an object at run-time and if necessary "downcast" it from a reference to a base class object to a reference to its actual type. A run-time type identification mechanism [14] has therefore been proposed for inclusion in the final standard. Note that Ada 9X already allows object types to be determined using the membership operator *in*.

There are a number of other issues which are still under consideration in C++ where the current language definition needs refinement. The definition of the lifetime of temporary objects is a typical example. Consider a class *String* which dynamically allocates memory to hold the value of the string which is later deallocated by the destructor. Given an overloaded "+" operator which performs concatenation and returns a *String* and a type conversion operator to *const char** which allows a *String* to be used wherever a string literal can be, a call such as *puts (a + b)* can fail to work correctly. The reason is that the "+" operator will need to create a temporary *String* object to hold its result. The type conversion operator is then applied, returning a pointer to the dynamically allocated memory. The temporary string is now no longer needed and a sufficiently aggressive compiler can delete it, resulting in the destructor deallocating the dynamic memory and *puts* being called with a dangling pointer as its argument.

Other problems arise from the low level of the base language. There is no bounds checking for array accesses in C++ as in C, but it is possible to define an *Array* class with a subscript operator with user-coded bounds checking. C and C++ programmers often complain that Ada's run-time checks reduce program efficiency, but as these checks are inserted by the compiler rather than the programmer they are at least amenable to optimisation. An *Array* class in C++ will perform bound checks even in situations where they can be statically guaranteed to be unnecessary, and this can result in a much less efficient program than the Ada equivalent.

The use of automatic type conversions is another source of problems. Although these are user-written functions, they are not called explicitly by the programmer. Instead, the compiler will insert invisible calls to these when it thinks it necessary. This can make debugging an activity full of interesting little surprises. User-defined type conversions are a useful feature, but they should not be called automatically; however, this is in keeping with C++'s heritage from C.

5.2. Templates.

Templates are becoming more widely available, but there are still many problems with them. They can be emulated using the standard C/C++ preprocessor, and this has resulted in the specification of a major feature of the language being based on a low-level macro facility which provides very little type safety. Unlike the generic features of Ada, there is no way to specify that the type supplied as a template parameter in C++ actually fulfils any desired semantic criteria. Any function or operator can be used with an unknown type T in a template definition, and it is only when an object is declared which instantiates T that the compiler can perform any type checking. If the actual type does not support the function or operator used, the compiler will then complain (usually citing an entirely erroneous position in the source file in the author's experience!); if however there is a function or operator with the correct name, it will be used even when it is completely inappropriate. In particular, strings are represented by pointers in C++ as in C; the comparison operator "<" is defined for pointers, so that a templated *sort* function when applied to an array of strings will compile successfully but will sort the strings by comparing their addresses rather than their contents. Special precautions must be taken to guard against this sort of situation which considerably complicate the design of templated classes and functions.

5.3. • Memory management problems.

C++ programs tend to rely heavily on dynamically-allocated memory. Typically a constructor will allocate memory using *new* and the destructor will delete it using *delete*. If there is insufficient memory, *new* will return a null pointer. In the absence of exceptions it is necessary to include explicit checks after constructing an object (since the constructor itself cannot return any result), something which is frequently not done. This is a major source of run-time errors in memory-intensive applications. Errors can also be made when deleting objects; if the destructor omits the call to *delete*, the program will suffer from "memory leaks" and eventually run out of memory. Deleting the same thing twice can also result in mysterious failures as the heap will normally become corrupted.

Another problem is that if an array of objects with destructors is created using *new*, it is necessary to use *delete [] X* rather than *delete X* to delete it as otherwise the destructor will only be called for the first object in the array. This again is a potent source of memory leak problems. It is not apparent to naive observers why it should be necessary to distinguish between the case of an array and a single element in this way, but it should be noted that the syntax and behaviour of *delete* has been evolving rapidly in recent language releases.

Garbage collection would be an ideal solution, but this is extremely difficult to implement for C++. Pointer arithmetic in C++ means that pointers can be adjusted to point to something other than the start of a block of memory, which makes it necessary to check to see if pointers refer to any position within a block. Worse still, the pointer can be moved beyond the end of the block, in which case the block appears to be free and a subsequent heap block appears to be in use. If garbage collection takes place before the pointer is adjusted back to a sensible value the effect will be disastrous.

5.4. Namespace pollution.

Namespace management is a major concern in C++. As more and more component libraries are developed, name clashes become more and more common; virtually every major component library contains a class called either *string* or *String*. Since all classes are declared globally (rather than within packages), this leads to major problems. In Ada, this would be a simple matter of qualifying type names with package names (e.g. *X.STRING* rather than *Y.STRING*). In C++ there is now a proposal to incorporate "namespace" declarations to resolve the problem [15] which is still under discussion by the standards committee. This proposal would allow classes to be enclosed in a package-like "namespace" block to remove the class names from the global name space.

A similar problem of namespace pollution might easily arise in connection with package names in Ada 9X as more and more reusable components become available. Naming conventions such as prefixing each package name with the name of the supplier can prevent name clashes occurring. However, child packages can also provide a convenient solution to this problem; for example, a software supplier could provide a (possibly empty) parent package which uses the supplier's name, and all other packages that they supply could be defined as child packages of the parent.

5.5. Standard libraries.

The lack of standard libraries for common data structures has proved to be a major problem in C++ which Ada 9X has not addressed. Object-oriented programming is all about developing reusable libraries of components. Some components are so common that virtually all libraries include them, largely because they are necessary building blocks for other components, and (at least in cases such as fundamental data structures) a standard library interface would greatly enhance portability. At present, most C++ applications aiming for portability are forced to re-invent the wheel as it is impossible to rely on a particular compiler providing any facilities other than input and output and the standard C functions. This tends to lead to large "all-purpose" libraries being developed, resulting in the problems described earlier in section 3.5. One of the major factors in making C as portable as it is is the availability of a set of common library functions defined by the language standard.

Stroustrup notes that "release 1.0 ... should have been delayed until a larger library including some simple classes such as singly and doubly linked lists, an associative array class, a range checked array class, and a simple string class could have been included. The absence of those led to everybody re-inventing the wheel and to an unnecessary diversity in the most fundamental classes" ([8], p. 295). Ada 9X is currently poised to fall into exactly the same trap, with only input and output packages and packages for low-level machine dependent facilities such as systems programming and interrupt handling being defined by the standard.

Ada 9X has also left the definition of TEXT_IO more or less unchanged from Ada 83. One of the problems with this is that it is aimed squarely at file-based I/O, and cannot be adapted by users wishing to modify it, for example for output to a particular screen region such as a window. C++ has defined a new "streams" library for input and output which makes the most of object-oriented design. Text formatting concerns are dealt with in the base class *ios* from which specific input and output streams are derived. Characters are written to and read from an instance of a class derived from *streambuf*. This makes it easy to retarget streams; simply derive a new buffer class from *streambuf* to display the characters on the screen in the correct way, and create a stream which uses this buffer. None of the facilities of TEXT_IO lend themselves to this kind of extension. Adapting TEXT_IO to write to a screen window involves formatting the data using PUT to produce a string and then displaying the string in an appropriate manner. Any other approach would involve reinventing a set of formatting routines for different data types with no possibility of reusing the formatting operations already present in the implementation of TEXT_IO.

6. Summary.

Both C++ and Ada 9X have their flaws; each lacks features that the other possesses although in both languages there are workarounds to compensate for the missing features. C++ is a language for adventurers; it is in a state of flux and it is insecure because it lacks Ada features like range checks. It also provides "state of the art" features such as multiple inheritance, which will help to increase our understanding of the subject. Ada 9X is conservatively designed; it is more secure than C++ but it has avoided including "state of the art" features which are not well understood. Anyone used to Ada would be infuriated by the "laissez faire" (or is it "caveat emptor"?) approach of C++; anyone used to C++ would likewise be outraged by Ada 9X's lack of constructors and destructors or multiple inheritance. Once you are used to the features available in a particular language, it is very hard to live without them again in another language even though workarounds can be used to provide similar capabilities.

Many of the shortcomings of C++ have been avoided in the design of Ada 9X. Some of the problems of C++, notably automatic type conversions and the low level of the base language, are problems "inherited" from C. The major shortcoming of C++ at present is the lack of exception handling facilities which have always been present in Ada, although it is hoped that this will soon be remedied in forthcoming compiler releases. Other problems such as the need to specify functions as being "virtual" as well as the need for constructs such as static members and friends, with complexities arising from interactions with templates and other features, result from the amalgamation of encapsulation and extensibility into a single construct. Ada packages allow extensibility to be considered separately from encapsulation in Ada 9X which results in a much simpler design in many ways.

The most serious omissions of Ada 9X (from the point of view of someone used to C++) are the lack of constructors and destructors, assignment overloading and multiple inheritance. Other differences such as the inability to define helper classes in the same way as in C++ will undoubtedly lead to different idiomatic design approaches in the two languages but are unlikely to reduce Ada 9X's expressive power.

Multiple inheritance is a difficult issue. It is probably too early to tell if other methods can adequately compensate for its absence; it is certainly too early to tell what the "correct" paradigm for multiple inheritance should be. As for constructors, destructors and user-defined assignment, the Ada 9X mapping team report that "we considered a general user-defined assignment and finalization capability. However, because of the large number of places within the language where implicit assignment or copy semantics are used ... user-defined assignment was determined to be too great an implementation burden if required of all Ada compilers." ([6], §3.2.4.1). However, this says nothing about constructors. C++ has come at the problem from the other end; that is, given constructors, destructors and user-defined assignment, how can exceptions be implemented? Early C++ implementations of exception handling indicate that the problem is not insuperable (merely very difficult!). Constructors and destructors can play a vital role in ensuring that objects are always in a valid state; their omission in Ada 9X leaves it up to the user to ensure object validity, which is likely to increase development and debugging costs.

Experience with C++ shows that it can quickly become very difficult to determine what operations are applicable to a given type at the bottom of an inheritance hierarchy several levels deep. Ensuring that coding standards are enforced from the very beginning will alleviate this problem, as will the use of automatic tools such as class browsers.

The major problem in Ada 9X is probably library support. It seems a great pity that a replacement for TEXT_IO was not introduced to make the most of the new features of Ada 9X along the lines of the C++ *iostream* classes. More seriously, Bjarne Stroustrup cites the lack of standard class libraries for C++ to be his worst mistake ([8], op.cit.). Ada 9X seems to be making exactly the same mistake. A lack of standard libraries will lead to a lot of wheels being continually reinvented in a variety of sizes and colours (and possibly even shapes!). This could easily lead to a lack of portability and also to over-generality and a lack of reusability, particularly if it tempts developers to produce monolithic Smalltalk-type designs as discussed earlier.

7. Conclusions.

The object-oriented programming facilities which C++ and Ada 9X have introduced into conventional procedural base languages are a welcome addition to the tools available to programmers concerned about issues of code reuse and maintenance. Although these facilities could be simulated by an assortment of programming tricks in the base languages involved, it would be impossible to force programmers to use such tricks consistently. Adding features such as those described in this paper to a language significantly increases its capabilities since they will be used as a matter of course by programmers, who in years to come will wonder how we ever used to manage without them (in much the same way as programmers now marvel at early machines without subroutine call instructions or hardware stack support).

C++ is a well-established and widely available language which has been instrumental in popularising the object-oriented programming paradigm. It suffers from a number of problems, partly due to its origins in C (a notoriously insecure language) and partly from its complexity. It is nevertheless an extremely influential and widely used object-oriented language. Its spread is fuelled by the wide availability of a range of cheap or free compilers and excellent development environments, as well as by a growing range of class libraries and bindings to existing systems.

Ada 9X, a relative latecomer to the object-oriented scene, suffers badly at the moment from a lack of availability even though it is at least as well-defined as C++. When Ada 9X compilers do become widely available, the Ada community will have to demonstrate that the same object-oriented design approaches can be used as in C++ and that the same application areas can be successfully addressed using Ada 9X, and that this can be done in a more secure way than in

C++. A range of libraries and bindings equivalent in scope to those available for C++ will need to be made available and standardised. Only then can Ada 9X become generally accepted. Most importantly, we can try to learn from the problems experienced in practice with C++ in order to avoid dealing with the same problems all over again when Ada 9X compilers are as widespread as C++ compilers are now.

References.

[1]   G. M. Birtwhistle, O-J Dahl, B Myrhaug & K. Nygaard, "SIMULA BEGIN". Auerbach 1973.

[2]   A. Goldberg & D. Robson, "Smalltalk-80: The Language and its Implementation". Addison-Wesley 1983.

[3]   B. Cox, "Object-Oriented Programming: An Evolutionary Approach". Addison-Wesley 1987.

[4]   B. Stroustrup, "The C++ Programming Language" (2nd edition). Addison-Wesley 1991.

[5]   M. A. Ellis & B. Stroustrup, "The Annotated C++ Reference Manual". Addison-Wesley 1990.

[6]   Ada 9X Project Office, "Ada 9X Mapping Document, vol. 1: Mapping Rationale". Intermetrics 1992.

[7]   Ada 9X Project Office, "Ada 9X Mapping Document, vol. 2: Mapping Specification". Intermetrics 1992.

[8]   B. Stroustrup, "A History of C++: 1979 – 1991". Proc. HOPL-II, SIGPLAN Notices 28 (3) pp. 271 – 297, 1993

[9]   A. Koenig & B. Stroustrup, "Exception Handling for C++". Journal of Object-Oriented Programming 3 (2) pp. 16 – 33, 1990.

[10]   J. Bengtsson, "C++, Without Exceptions". Telia Research, Luleå, Sweden, 1992.

[11]   K. E. Gorlen, S. M. Orlow & P. S. Plexico, "Data Abstraction and Object-Oriented Programming in C++". John Wiley 1990.

[12]   B. Meyer, "Object-Oriented Software Construction". Prentice Hall 1988.

[13]   E. Siedewitz, "Object-Oriented Programming with Mixins in Ada". Ada Letters XII (2) pp. 76 – 90, 1992.

[14]   B. Stroustrup and D. Lenkov, "Run-Time Type Identification for C++". The C++ Report, March 1992.

[15]   B. Stroustrup, "Name Space Management in C++ (revised)". ANSI X3J16 working paper WG21/N0262, 1993.

High Integrity Ada: Principles and Problems

John A McDermid

York Software Engineering Limited
and
University of York
Heslington, York YO1 5DD, UK

Abstract There is increasing use of Ada in High Integrity, especially Safety Critical, applications, but the requirements of these applications are often in conflict with using the full range of features of the Ada language. The aim of this paper is to illuminate the issues in developing Ada software to the high levels of integrity required for such applications, and to show the 'state of the art' in developing and assessing such systems, including the use of Ada subsets and of static analysis and verification techniques. Much of the work on which this paper is based was carried out as part of a study for the MoD; the paper concludes with an outline of the recommendations to the MoD on the use of Ada in high integrity applications and a discussion of some open issues.

1   Introduction

There is increasing use of Ada in High Integrity, especially Safety Critical, applications, e.g. civil and military aircraft systems and aero-engine controllers (FADECs). The requirements which these systems have to meet so that they can be certified and released into service are stringent, and are in conflict with using the full range of features of the Ada language. For example, the use of full Ada in Safety Critical Defence Applications is in conflict with the requirement to verify systems to the standards required by Interim Defence Standard (IDS) 00-55 [1], both at the current state of verification technology and at a more fundamental level as certain aspects of the language do not have well-defined semantics.

The aim of this paper is to illuminate the issues in using Ada in Safety Critical applications. It builds on *A Study of High Integrity Ada* carried out by York Software Engineering (YSE) Limited and BAe Defence Limited (Military Aircraft Division) for the Ministry of Defence (MoD) under contract SLS31c/73, and research work undertaken in the University of York. The primary aim of the study was to provide recommendations on the policy which the MoD should adopt *vis a vis* the use of Ada in High Integrity Applications in the light of the requirements of IDS 00-55 and IDS 00-56[1] [2] which set out the standards for developing software in Safety Critical systems, and the principles for hazard analysis of Safety Critical programmable electronic systems, respectively. The aim of much of the research work in York is to bring non-functional program properties, such as timing and resource usage within the realms of static analysis, i.e. to make it possible to determine these properties analytically, rather than through testing. However we also address some work concerned with formal development of Ada programs.

---

[1] IDS 00-56 has been under revision, and it has been reissued in draft form, since the study was completed. The work decribed here was based on the 1991 standard; it is believed that all the observations made here are compatible with the new standard, but the primary study reports make some observations on IDS 00-56 which are no longer valid, assuming that the current draft is indicative of the eventual content of the new standard.

1.1   Technical Background

The detailed technical requirements for showing that a High Integrity software (controlled) system is fit to be deployed vary from industry to industry, but there is a general requirement to be able to define precisely the behaviour of such a system prior to deployment, by static analysis, verification, dynamic analysis (testing) or a combination of these means. In general it is necessary to be able to characterise behaviour in four 'domains':

- functionality;

- timing;

- resource usage;

- failure behaviour.

In practice, failure behaviour may simply be a special case of the functionality domain, being concerned with the functions to be executed when failures of 'peripherals' occur, although it may be more complex if there is a requirement to show tolerance to processor or software 'failures'. Much work on static analysis and verification concentrates on the functional issues; in the High Integrity Ada study, we tried to take a more balanced view of these issues, and the research work in the University focuses more on the non-functional than functional properties.

Differing industries have widely varying standards which set out specific guidelines for choosing an appropriate balance of static analysis, verification and dynamic testing techniques to show that a system behaves as required. Oversimplifying to make the point, the civil aerospace guidelines, RTCA DO-178B [3], are firmly based on the principle that demonstration of correct program behaviour should be undertaken by testing. On the other hand IDS 00-55 (which is applied in military aerospace and other defence projects) places the greatest stress on static analysis and verification (sometimes referred to as 'program proving'), although it also requires extensive testing to be carried out. Thus, if we are to apply IDS 00-55, we are concerned with the ability to analyse statically and to verify the functional, timing, resource usage and failure behaviour of programs.

1.2   Overview of *A Study of High Integrity Ada*

A Study of High Integrity Ada (hereinafter referred to as the study) considered current practice, available and emerging technology, as well as investigating the requirements of the standards; the focus was on static analysis, and we exclude testing from this paper. The study produced a number of results, including:

1   a definition of a set of criteria for assessing the suitability of a programming language, or subset, for use in High Integrity applications;

2   a definition of an Ada subset which met the criteria;

3   identification of static analysis and verification technology that could be applied to the toolset;

4   identification of issues which need to be addressed in carrying out a hazard analysis of development processes and toolsets, and the management of 'sub-ideal' processes;

5   a set of recommendations for a policy statement by the MoD covering language subsets, toolsets, education and training, and other actions on demonstrators and standards;

6   a set of recommendations for further work by the MoD covering long term standardisation, tool development, etc.

This paper summarises most of the issues listed above, but completely excludes point 4, on processes, toolsets and related issues, e.g. the hazard analysis of toolsets. The latter is a difficult issue; it is clearly appropriate to analyse the 'indirect hazards' which tools can pose to applications software, especially the effects that a compilation system can have on integrity. However, this is felt to be a research issue, as some insight is required to determine the most appropriate way to assess indirect hazards. We do not treat this point at length in the paper, although it is an important topic.

1.3 Organisation of the Paper

The rest of the paper is organised as follows. Section 2 discusses the issue of language requirements for High Integrity applications and how various Ada subsets meet these requirements. It also addresses the state of the art in analysis technology, covering the four key aspects of program behaviour, and the issue of compilation integrity. Section 3 outlines the recommendations made to the MoD. Section 4 considers practical problems that arise out of the state of current technology, and identifies some longer term research issues. Finally it gives some general conclusions regarding applications of Ada in High Integrity applications. Where appropriate we complement the results of the study by indicating relevant research and development work being undertaken at YSE and in the University.

2 Ada Subsets and Analysis Technology

One of the major contributions of the study was the definition of a set of criteria for assessing the suitability of a programming language, or subset, for use in High Integrity applications. We outline these requirements and identify some of the key properties of a suitable Ada subset, and then give an overview of current technology to indicate what static analysis and verification can be done now, or will be feasible in the near future.

2.1 Language Requirements and Ada Subsets

We discuss language requirements, outline the subset we identified in the study, compare this subset with SPARK Ada, and make some observations about a possible subset of Ada9X.

2.1.1 Language Requirements

We identified five basic requirements for a programming language for High Integrity applications:

L1   A high integrity software language must be well-understood, simple to understand, simple to learn, simple to use, simple to implement, and simple to reason about.

L2   A high integrity software language must provide features appropriate to that application domain.

L3   Prior to execution, it must be possible to predict the following properties of a program written in a high integrity software language:

— functionality;

— timing;

— resource usage;

— failure behaviour.

L4   It must be possible to verify that a program written in a high integrity software language is correct with respect to a specification expressed in a formal notation.

L5   There must be a high level of assurance in a high integrity software language's compilation system and associated tools.

Whilst these requirements are influenced by IDS 00-55 and IDS 00-56, they are also broadly accepted in other domains, e.g. civil aerospace, although there is less willingness to accept the relevance of L4 outside the defence arena (e.g. they are admitted, but not advocated, by RTCA DO-178B). However, there is evidence that formal methods are being applied successfully in a number of critical applications in Europe and North America [4]. It should also be noted that these requirements are, to some extent, in conflict, e.g. ease of use means that the language should be highly expressive, and this may act against verifiability. Thus, in defining a high integrity software language it is necessary to make trade-offs. The nature of the trade-offs are not 'black and white', so there is some room for value judgements in defining a subset, and the scale of 'the most appropriate' subset will indubitably change as static analysis and verification technology matures. It is also to be expected that an extended subset will be defined to incorporate features of Ada9X, see Section 2.1.4 below.

2.1.2 The YSE Subset

Our subset and the rationale for choosing the subset are given in [6]. As is the norm for subset definitions, we characterise our subset in relation to the full Ada language in terms of the major exclusions and restrictions. The restrictions are not just syntactic, and their enforcement requires semantic analysis. The major exclusions are:

- anonymous types;
- discriminated types;
- access types;
- derived types;
- aliasing;
- recursion;
- use clauses;
- tasks;
- generics.

The major areas of restrictions are:

- all constraints must be static;
- no default expressions are allowed;
- functions must not have any side effects;
- there are limitations on the placement of return statements;
- only some loop constructions are admissible;
- pre-defined exceptions must not be raised.

Note that our subset permits overloading, user-defined exception handling and the use of Chapter 13 features.

The subset of Ada outlined above is, we believe, the largest which fully meets our requirements for a high integrity software language, given current analysis and verification technology, and it is certainly larger than any of the Ada subsets mentioned in Section 2.2. We suggest that it balances the requirement for simplicity (L1), particularly simplicity of reasoning, and expressive power (L2) in the most appropriate manner. It is both predictable across the domains of functionality, timing and resource (memory) usage (L3), and verifiable (L4) at the current state-of-the-art. The state of the art in commercially available and research tools indicate that a range of high integrity tools could be constructed to support the use of our subset (L5).

2.1.3 The YSE Subset and SPARK Ada

The best known Ada subset in industrial use is SPARK [5], defined and commercially supported by Program Validation Limited (PVL). Our conclusions were that SPARK was somewhat over-restrictive, but that it was an appropriate language in terms of our requirements. In other words SPARK is within the 'grey area' of trade-offs between expressive power and analysability but, in our view, errs towards analysability more than is necessary. Nonetheless it is clear that SPARK is the closest approach to meeting our language requirements of any commercially supported language. Technically our subset [6] is more regular than SPARK, e.g. in the area of visibility. It includes user defined exceptions (although it is still necessary to show that pre-defined exceptions cannot be raised). Our subset also allows overloading, which is particularly useful, e.g. in defining application specific arithmetic functions.

2.1.4 A Subset of Ada9X

Our focus was primarily on Ada83 and, of course, a subset of Ada 83 is also a subset of Ada9X. However there is some benefit to be gained from defining an extended subset for Ada9X, although the extensions are not large. We believe that it is possible and appropriate to include generics and a restricted form of tasking allowing communication only via protected objects. Ada9X generics are analysable (in Ada 83 they are not; the substantive difference is in the contract model) and protected objects give an analysable form of concurrency. All Ada83 subsets exclude derived types, because of difficulties they introduce for analysis — and this would suggest that we would have to preclude the object oriented features of Ada9X, although this is arguably one of the language's strongest (most popular) features. It may be possible to restrict the situations in which derived types (inheritance) can be used, and thus admit some of the object oriented features. This is an open issue, but benefit would certainly accrue from a more complete study of this issue.

2.2 Analysis and Verification

There are a number of commercially available static analysis and verification tools based on Ada and Ada subsets, and a larger number of research projects. Again the SPARK Examiner [7] is well-known in the UK; however we focus here on other, less well-known, developments including those in the USA. Our aim is to give an overview of current capability; a full review is beyond the scope of this paper. The interested reader is referred to [6] for more details. We discuss systems in terms of the classification of properties laid out under requirement L3.

2.2.1 Functionality

We briefly review a number of existing systems, and some systems under development, comparing and contrasting the styles of the systems.

Systems for investigating functionality are typified by the SPARK Examiner. The Examiner supports static analysis of programs, e.g. it determines the flow of information through programs, and enables anomalies to be detected such as data being read before it is written. This is a useful quality assurance tool, but it should be noted that these anomalies do not always represent flaws in the program — the data may be set by a memory mapped hardware device, so the 'anomaly' simply reflects proper program behaviour in this case. Thus judgement is required in interpreting the results from such tools.

The SPARK Examiner also supports formal specification of program behaviour by means of annotations, in a form of predicate logic couched in Ada-like syntax. The annotations can be used for a number of purposes, most commonly to show input-output relations, i.e. to specify what outputs should be produced for a given set of inputs. These facilities enable low-level program verification to be carried out, i.e. it is possible to verify the correlation between annotations and the program, using the Examiner. The term 'low-level' implies that the annotations are in terms of program constructs not more abstract properties, and may not directly reflect the program or system requirements. In use, the software engineer submits annotated programs to the tool, the tool extracts proof obligations, i.e. putative theorems which need to be proven to show that the program satisfies the annotations, then the user attempts to discharge the obligations with assistance from a proof tool. This is very much the classical style of program verification, as typified by systems such as Gypsy developed in the 1970's. Note that the proofs are only partial; they say that the program satisfies its specifications *if* it terminates, but they don't show termination.

In the USA there are several interesting developments — we mention two which exhibit quite markedly different styles. Odyssey Research Associates (ORA) at Ithaca are developing a system known as Penelope [8] based on a mechanisation of the wp-calculus [9]. In the wp-calculus, a post-condition is given saying what state the program is intended to establish, when it has completed executing. The post-condition will restrict the values of the program variables and its outputs. The wp-calculus gives rules for 'pushing the post-condition back through the program' to calculate a weakest pre-condition (hence the term wp) which is the weakest constraint which can be made on the program variables and inputs when the program is invoked in order to guarantee that it will satisfy its post-condition once it has terminated. If the wp is TRUE, then the program will always satisfy its post-condition, but normally the pre-condition expresses validity constraints on inputs, e.g. the acceptable (expected) range of values from a sensor. Penelope supports a form of program verification based on the wp-calculus applied to a significant (and growing) subset of Ada which includes user-defined exceptions, and experimental work is being done on tasks and generics. One of the interesting aspects of Penelope is that it is highly interactive, and incremental. If one gives a post-condition and an outline of the program structure, e.g. an IF statement and the conditional expression, Penelope will calculate the pre-conditions automatically. Thus it is possible to develop programs and the associated proofs incrementally and interactively. This is a much more intuitive way to develop and verify programs than the classical style, but the approach is only effective if the programs can be broken down into small modules.

Computational Logic Incorporated (CLInc) are developing support for a language know as AVA [10] — A Verifiable Ada. Like Penelope, the aim is to work towards support for a large subset of Ada, although the style of the system is very different. One of the key concerns in developing a verification system of the nature discussed here is whether or not the tools correctly reflect the language semantics. The approach used by the AVA team is to make the encoding of the proof system in their verification tools correlate as directly as possible with the language semantics (in this case a formal operational semantics). The AVA tools are being developed as part of a research project at CLInc, and will probably end up as a classical form of verification system, supporting a subset similar to SPARK. At the time we saw the system (May 1992) the tool development was at a very early stage, and certainly was not complete enough to verify anything other than very simple programs.

There is benefit to be gained from verifying the compliance between relatively low-level specifications or annotations, and programs, e.g. it is possible to verify safety properties expressed in terms of the program state (variables). However, much greater benefit can be gained if programs are verified against a much more abstract specification, which is much closer to the requirements, or problem domain, as there is much less opportunity for undetected error in writing the formal specification, e.g. misrepresenting the safety requirements. However, if high-level formal specifications are given, it is necessary to develop the program within the formal framework if the benefits of the mathematical rigour are not to be lost. This type of development process is usually known as formal refinement. Refinement is not a panacea, but it does offer an opportunity for formally relating programs to higher level specifications. At YSE work is being undertaken on the development of a tool known as ZETA, which provides support for formal development of SPARK programs from Z specifications. ZETA is an extension of YSE's Z support tool, known as CADiZ [11], which provides static checking of Z specifications, and an interactive facility for investigating and manipulating specifications, e.g. calculating pre-conditions.

The method supported by ZETA involves stepwise refinement, using an approach known as a 'formal web' for representing refinement steps. The method [12] was developed at the DRA Malvern and is based on a combination of Morgan's refinement calculus [13] and Knuth's ideas of literate programming [14]. This approach offers the possibility of refining from more abstract specifications, and thus overcoming some of the limitations of existing tools, although this introduces other technical problems, e.g. verifying the mapping between some abstract data representation and an Ada data type. This style of development also gives the opportunity to develop critical parts of the program formally, and other parts in a systematic, but informal, manner. This potentially offers high levels of assurance, at reduced cost, by focusing on those aspects of the program where the formal approach gives the highest returns for effort expended.

In practice, fully formal development of programs is difficult, and has not been successfully achieved except for small programs. All the systems described above have technical limitations, above and beyond issues of scalability, in the size of subset supported, completeness of the tools, or other areas. Thus satisfaction of IDS 00-55 is feasible for small programs, but there are difficulties encountered in applying any of the available approaches in the large. Also the diversity of the tools suggests that either there is no 'best way' of formally developing programs or, perhaps more likely, that the technology is insufficiently mature for the most appropriate approach to have been identified. There is some merit in both interpretations, and we can expect program verification systems to evolve, and different styles of system to be advocated, for some time to come.

2.2.2 Timing

In order to evaluate timing properties of programs we need two complementary pieces of information: the worst case execution times (WCETs) of the fragments of code which are executed by the system between scheduling points, and the policy implemented by the scheduler, for determining the order in which theses code fragments are executed. Modern scheduling theory [15] makes it possible to implement quite sophisticated scheduling policies, however most practical real-time systems use static cyclic scheduling, and system level timing properties can be derived from those of the code fragments, simply by adding together the WCETs of the code fragments executed in a given cycle.

Timing properties of programs are normally determined by dynamic analysis, however it is possible to evaluate timing properties of programs and systems by means of static analysis, specifically WCETs are evaluated by static analysis of code fragments. The benefit of such an approach is the ability to determine the worst case with a high degree of confidence (although it does rely on correct loop bound annotations), rather than relying on the test engineer to identify particular data which will evoke worst case behaviour of the program. A potential disadvantage is the fact that static analysis may produce pessimistic results unless they can do sophisticated semantic analysis of the programs, thus limiting (or negating) its value. However practical program timing analysis tools can produce results which are within 20% of the actual worst case (i.e. no more than 120% of the actual worst case), which is on a par with figures that can be achieved by testing.

Precise WCETs can only be derived once information is available at the object level, i.e. instruction numbers and orderings are known. However analysis purely at the object level produces pessimistic results as already noted — paths through the programs which are syntactically feasible are infeasible due to the semantics of the source program, but this is not apparent at object level. Thus combined source and object analysis is required to produce good predictions of program timing. Work undertaken by the University and YSE for the European Space Agency has resulted in some prototype tools [16] which support this form of static program timing analysis for a subset of Ada much larger than SPARK, and including an implementation of Ada 9X protected objects. Language features such as user defined exceptions can also be handled [17], so it is possible to handle the subset defined in the study (see section 2.1) although these mechanisms are not currently implemented in practical tools. It is also possible to deal with some of the more complex features of modern processors, e.g. pipelines [18], without getting unduly pessimistic results, although developments in modern processor technology, including caches, continue to pose new challenges.

It is now technically possible to perform static analysis of timing properties of realistic programs [19], although the application of this technology is still very much at the experimental stage. There seems no reason, however, why there should not be a progressive increase in the use of static analysis of timing properties, as the benefits of the approach become more widely realised, and more analysis tools become available. Indeed YSE are currently investigating the application of this form of tool for a major aerospace company, and the University are carrying out research into the development of such tools, again with backing from the aerospace industry.

2.2.3 Resource Usage

As with timing, resource, especially memory, usage is typically assessed by means of testing. In practice a key capability is to be able to evaluate stack usage, as the bounds on stack space are often not apparent from the program structure, and catastrophic failures may occur if a stack overflows physical memory. In principle the program timing analysis mechanisms can be adapted to evaluate resource usage, and we have experimentally validated this by extending the tools described in [16][2]. The general comments made about timing analysis apply to resource usage also, but it can be seem clearly here that we must eliminate (unbounded) recursion and the use of data structures which require heap storage from programs if we are to analyse them.

If one considers system level, rather than program level, analysis then it is also necessary to consider bus utilisation, etc. Work has been done in this area, but it is beyond the scope of this paper.

2.2.4 Failure Behaviour

For certification or clearance of Safety Critical systems it is usually necessary to carry out safety analysis, including determining the behaviour of the system in the presence of failures. Where software plays a key role in preserving safety, then it is necessary to apply equivalent analysis to the software. Responses to certain classes of failure, e.g. those outside the computing system, often appear as part of the functional specification[3]. In this case, requirements for the software to detect and recover from external failures can reduce to analysis of functionality. Functional verification can then be used to demonstrate the role of the software in achieving safety. However, this is not sufficient to show how the program will respond to internal failures due either to hardware faults affecting the program or residual design errors, and it is relevant to consider other ways of performing safety analysis.

It is desirable for the software safety analysis to be carried out using techniques similar to those applied to other technologies, in order that the analysis results can be integrated to provide a complete system-level safety analysis. Classical techniques include: Fault Tree Analysis (FTA) [20] which works back from a known hazard to determine the possible causes of the hazard; and Failure Modes and Effects Analysis (FMEA) [21] which works forwards from known causes to determine their effects.

It is possible to adapt classical failure analysis techniques, e.g. fault trees, to software safety analysis and it has been shown that these are technically equivalent to the wp-calculus [9], under certain assumptions [22]. Pragmatically the application of software fault trees is equivalent to functional verification, directed at the hazards not the normal post-condition (i.e. normal program behaviour). Thus these techniques can be used to provide formally sound, hazard directed, analyses. These ideas were first applied to Ada by Leveson and her colleagues [23]. Some experimental work has also been done in York on the development of tools to support fault tree analysis of Ada subset programs, and their application to a number of aerospace examples [24].

This work is more tentative than that on static timing analysis, but there is some evidence that it is possible to apply the classical safety analysis techniques to programs, and thereby to provide evidence that can form an overall part of the safety case. It should be noted that the status of such technology *vis a vis* IDS 00-55 and RTCA DO-178B is unclear — it is not mentioned explicitly by either standard, yet it seems relevant as a way of producing a unified safety case. Further, it overlaps with functional verification, at least for certain classes of failure mode. Additional study is needed to determine the circumstances (if any) where such technology forms an effective part of a High Integrity system development method.

---

[2] This work has not been published; it involved evaluating stack usage of programs taregtted at an MC68020 by means of object level analysis.

[3] In our experience, it is common for such requirements to appear in the functional specifications.

2.3   Compilation Integrity

Concern is often expressed about the use of Ada (and other high level languages) in developing safety critical systems, as the language provides a 'barrier' between the software engineer and what is 'really happening' in the machine — and clearly it is the object programs which ultimately need to be verified against requirements, or at least shown to be equivalent to the source code where that has been verified. The normal advantages of high level languages do, of course, aid the process of developing clear and intelligible code, but they can hinder the process of gaining the ultimate assurance in the executing code. In principle, at least, there is a trade-off between language complexity and ease of assurance, as the more complex (sophisticated or expressive) the language becomes, the greater the 'gap' between source and object program.

The main technical concern over compilation integrity is the fact Ada compilers are very complex, often at least an order of magnitude larger than the application they are compiling — or even worse in some Safety Critical applications! Most compilers implement very subtle and sophisticated optimisations[4], whereas the applications are typically much simpler, e.g. they may, for the most part, simply implement Boolean logic functions. Thus the compiler may be a significant source of unreliability, and it is necessary to verify that the compiler preserves the semantics of the Ada programs, or more strictly that the compilations used to build the application which is deployed preserve the integrity of the application. This leads to a requirement to demonstrate the integrity of the compiler.

IDS 00-55 requires that the compiler is formally specified and verified[5] to the same degree of rigour as safety critical application code. Such formal developments are beyond the state of the art (by some margin) due to the complexity of Ada compilers. However for simpler languages, compilation integrity can be demonstrated by applying static analysis technology to the results of particular compilations, e.g. as has been done for PLM/86 on Sizewell B [25]. RTCA DO-178B takes a rather more pragmatic stance, relying primarily on testing in source terms to show that the compilation is satisfactory, but requiring that special measures are taken where the compiler generates code which is not manifest in the source, e.g. array bound checks. An interesting possibility is the combination of static analysis and testing to ensure path coverage of both source and object. In practice, most compiler (or compilation) verification takes place by a combination of testing and manual inspection of object code.

This problem is exacerbated with Ada, as the standard admits no subsets. Thus, for example, SPARK programs still have to be compiled through a full Ada compiler, although much of the complexity is not needed for the subset. Thus, in principle, we would expect a SPARK compiler (or a compiler for a similar size subset) to be simpler, and of higher integrity. It should also be noted that this is not just an issue of size — it is likely that simpler compilation strategies could be used, without producing unacceptable code. The Safety and Security Annex of the Ada 9X draft standard allows subsets[6], and also requires the provision of mapping information which will help compilation verification and the timing and resource analysis outlined above. Thus Ada 9X seems to be a better basis for gaining high integrity compilers, but there are some commercial issues, see Section 4.

2.4   Summary

It is clear that there is a reasonably good understanding of how to verify (statically analyse) functional, timing and resource properties of programs, and there is an emerging understanding of the issues of handling failure behaviour. There are some

---

[4] We are informed that one of the best-known commercially available Ada compilers uses 42 optimisations, whose application is determined heuristically.

[5] An alternative is quoted, but this seems to amount to verifying the compilation!.

[6] This has been a matter of some debate, and it is not clear whether or not this will be seen as a commercially viable option by compiler vendors.

workable tools, and the technology can be applied to small programs. However the technology is fragmented; the language subsets for which there exist timing analysers are different to those for which functional verification technology exists, and so on. At present the developer of High Integrity Ada programs has to do a lot of work to draw together a viable toolset, and worse has to repeat analysis work as, for example, the analysis of control flow in a program underlies all the major verification activities, and is the basis for systematic testing. There is a clear need for a more concerted effort on tool development, and on integration of these different technologies both to produce efficient toolsets, and to ease the burden on the software developer.

3   Recommendations from the Study

Our recommendations fell into three main areas: issues to be addressed in a policy statement; other short term recommendations; long term issues. We recommended the publication of a policy statement because we believed that the interaction between policies, e.g. the preference for Ada and IDS 00-55, is not clear, and due to the pragmatic difficulties of conforming to IDS 00-55 as it stands. It is intended that the policy statement would be supported with detailed guidance, based on the findings of the study.

Our recommendations identified five main issues to be covered by the policy statement:

R1   The MoD should require all suppliers to use languages and associated toolsets which satisfy the requirements set out in section 2.1.

R2   The MoD should require all suppliers to comply with the Ada subset defined in the study, or show why the language they propose satisfies the requirements at least as well; it was explicitly noted that SPARK satisfies this criterion.

R3   The MoD should require all suppliers to use a minimal acceptable toolset or show why the toolset they propose is of the same or better capability than the minimal acceptable.

R4   The MoD should require all suppliers to provide a 'safety case' for their development process and toolset, to show that they have achieved the necessary integrity, including having ways of dealing with flawed or limited tools.

R5   The MoD should require all suppliers to use staff qualified according to the guidelines set out in the BCS Industry Structure Model Safety Critical Systems sub-stream [26].

A rationale for these recommendations is given in the report. Two points are worth noting here. The definition of languages and toolsets is intended to remove uncertainty about how to interpret standards, and to give some focus to the otherwise disparate tools market. R5 is included as we believe that the skills of the development staff are probably the most significant factor in achieving integrity, yet this fact is not properly recognised in IDS 00-55 (although it was in a pre-publication draft).

The other two short term recommendations were:

R6   The MoD should update IDS 00-55 and IDS 00-56 to take into account the difficulties in applying the standards which were identified by the study.

R7   The MoD should fund demonstrator projects to give clear evidence on the efficacy of the standards, and to help establish acceptable ways of interpreting and applying the standards.

To some extent, both these recommendations have been overtaken by events, as the MoD started programmes to address these issues before the study finished.

The longer term recommendations were:

R8   The MoD should provide stimulus for tool development, as market demands alone are inadequate to lead to the development of tools satisfying IDS 00-55.

R9   The MoD should work with others, e.g. the DTI and CEC, to establish a centre for assessing processes and toolsets for their compliance with the requirements of the standards; there is an analogy here with the security evaluation facilities.

R10   The MoD should work with others, e.g. the SERC, to foster the establishment of appropriate education and training, e.g. post-experience MSc, and progressively require graduation from these courses as a prerequisite for filling roles identified in the standards, e.g. Independent Safety Assessor.

R11   The MoD should (seek to) influence the wider standardisation community, and seek to ensure convergence between their standards, and those in other nations and industries.

The aim of these recommendations is to increase the ease with, and extent to, which industry can conform to the MoD's requirements, whilst reducing the gulf between MoD requirements and those in the wider marketplace, thus leading to more cost-effective developments. Clearly the above recommendations represent a compromise between principles and pragmatism, but we believe they offer a realistic way of improving standards, without the MoD ending up with unique, and hence expensive, requirements and standards.

Finally, it should be stressed that *these are our recommendations to the MoD, not the policy of the MoD.*

4   Practical Problems and Conclusions

We briefly summarise our main findings, and draw out some broader issues for consideration. The requirements of IDS 00-55 can be satisfied in the context of Ada, in principle, in the small; however, there are difficulties of scaling the technology, and the application of static analysis to non-functional properties, such as timing, is still at the experimental stage. Nonetheless we have a basis on which to build, and more effective tools can be produced if the market conditions are suitable, or the MoD can stimulate the market. We have made some recommendations which, if implemented, will, we believe, ease the transition to more complete and cost-effective satisfaction of the requirements of IDS 00-55 and IDS 00-56. We have also recommended that the MoD place more stress on individual skills and capabilities as this is probably the greatest determinant of integrity, in practice[7].

Some slightly more general observations should be made. The above analysis shows that the state of tool support for developing High Integrity programs in Ada is less than ideal — this raises the question of whether or not other languages offer a better basis for such developments. A number of aerospace companies[8] have their own proprietary development systems which avoid some of the difficulties noted above, and have proven effective in practice. Generally these are 'low-level high-level' languages, and give some of the advantages of languages such as Ada, but without introducing the difficulties of compilation verification as they are much 'closer to the machine'. Arguably these are a better place at which to start than Ada, but their proprietary nature precludes them from being a basis for a widely supported language standard and toolset. This reinforces our view that an agreement to use a specific Ada subset, together with the acceptance that it is legitimate to produce subset compilers and thereby regain some of the advantages of the proprietary solutions, is a crucial factor in achieving a widely available toolset for the development of High Integrity software.

We now conclude with some open questions, many of which address the practicality of our views on the production of a widely available toolset for the development of high integrity software. These are the 'problems' in the title — they represent problems to which we do not, as yet, have adequate solutions.

---

[7] Arguably 'safety culture' is the most crucial factor; however we do not claim to be able to define how a safety culture can be established or assessed, so we did not address this issue in our recommendations.

[8] And perhaps others in other industries, but we are not aware of any.

One of the biggest practical problems facing the developers and assessors of High Integrity software is to do with compiler complexity, and reliability. There is a strong technical case for building a high integrity subset compiler, e.g. based on SPARK, although commercial issues tend to mitigate against this, i.e. the market for such compilers is perhaps 1% of the overall Ada market. How should this be resolved? Can a satisfactory solution be found in the context of Ada 9X?

There is technical and commercial advantage to be gained from building tools around an agreed language subset. SPARK is the best established subset, but it has limitations, some of which can be removed by extending static analysis and verification technology to work in the context of Ada 9X. Is it practical to get agreement to such a language to give a focus for tool development? Would such a subset be agreed by a large enough part of the relevant industries (Defence and aerospace are probably the key industries) that such a development would be commercially viable?

One problem with current technology is how to deal with large scale systems. How can the technology be developed to make it scale? Is a concerted (world-wide) effort needed on this problem — arguably the North Americans are far ahead in verification technology, but they are unlikely to want to support UK standards?

The skills required to develop systems using the available analysis technology are not widespread. How can the gulf between available technology and skills be reduced/eliminated? Should there be greater sponsorship for post-graduate courses? Can professional bodies such as the IEE and BCS, or industry bodies such as the SBAC and EEA, act as catalysts for improving the quality of education and training?

There is a further problem — the principles adopted by many standards are promulgated on the basis of dogma, or faith, not hard evidence of the efficacy of the techniques. How do we gain evidence that will enable us to select methods for their proven effectiveness, especially where we might expect zero errors in a system's operational life? Perhaps this is the most major issue as this is a critical part of the data which the community needs in order to put High Integrity software development on a proper engineering footing.

5   Acknowledgements

The study which formed the basis for this paper was undertaken by a number of people at YSE, the University of York and BAe Defence Limited (Military Aircraft Division), funded by the MoD under contract SLS31c/73. Special thanks go to Brian Jepson, Charles Forsyth, Andy Hutcheon, David Jordan and Ian Wand for their contributions to the study, and to the MoD reviewers for their helpful, insightful (and at times taxing) comments and criticism. David Jordan also provided some very helpful comments on an earlier version of this paper.

Thanks also go to the staff at PVL, TACS, ORA in Ithaca and Ottawa, CLInc in Austin, Texas, SRI International in Menlo Park, California and the Aerospace Corporation in Los Angeles for their help in the conduct of the study. Much of the research work referred to has been undertaken within the High Integrity Systems Engineering (HISE) and Real-Time Systems (RTS) groups in York. I am happy to acknowledge the work of Alan Burns and Andy Wellings who lead the RTS group, and all the staff in the RTS and HISE groups who have contributed to the development of the ideas and tools referred to above.

6   References

[1]   Ministry of Defence, *The Procurement of Safety Critical Software in Defence Equipment*, Interim Defence Standard 00-55, April 1991.

[2]   Ministry of Defence, *Hazard Analysis and Safety Classification of the Computer and Programmable Electronic Elements of Defence Equipment*, Interim Defence Standard 00-56, April 1991.

[3]   RTCA/EUROCAE, *Software Considerations in Airborne Systems and Equipment Certification*, DO-178B, 1993.

[4]   D Craigen, S Gerhart, T Ralston, *An International Survey of Industrial Applications of Formal Methods*, NIST GCR 93/626, National Institute of Science and Technology, 1993.

[5]   T J Jennings, B A Carre, *A Subset of Ada for Formal Verification*, Ada User Vol. 9, pp 121-126, 1989.

[6]   A D Hutcheon, B J Jepson, D T Jordan, J A McDermid, I C Wand, *Analysis of Ada Programs*, Report SLS31c/73-2-D, YSE and BAe Defence, 1993[9].

[7]   B A Carre, J Garnsworthy, *Experiences with SPARK and its support tool, the Examiner*, in Proceedings of Ada UK International Conference, 1990.

[8]   Odyssey Research Associates, *Penelope Volume I: Collected Papers in Ada Verification*, ORA, Itahaca, 1989-1990.

[9]   E W Dijkstra, *A Discipline of Programming*, Prentice Hall, 1976.

[10]   M K Smith, *The AVA Reference Manual*, Computational Logic, Inc., 1992.

[11]   D Jordan, J A McDermid, I Toyn, *CADiZ — Computer Aided Design in Z*, in Z User Workshop, Oxford (1990), J E Nicholls (ed), Springer Verlag 1991.

[12]   C T Sennett, *Demonstrating the Compliance of Ada Programs with Z Specifications*, Defence Research Agency, Malvern 1991.

[13]   C C Morgan, *Programming from Specifications*, Prentice Hall, 1990.

[14]   D E Knuth, *Literate Programming*, Computer Journal, Vol. 27, No. 2, 1984.

[15]   A Burns, *Scheduling hard real-time systems : a review*, Software Engineering Journal, Vol. 6, No. 3, 1991

[16]   C H Forsyth, *Implementation of the Worst Case Execution Analyser*, YSE Report: ESTEC Contract No. 9198/90/NL/SF, Task 8, Vol. E, 1992.

[17]   R Chapman, A Burns, A J Wellings, *Worst-case timing analysis of exception handling in Ada*, in Proceedings of Ada UK, IOS Press, 1993.

[18]   N Zhang, A Burns, M Nicholson, *Pipelined Processors and Worst Case Execution Times,* YCS 198, Department of Computer Science, University of York, 1993.

[19]   C Bailey, E Fyfe, A Burns, A J Wellings, *The Olympus Attitude and Orbital Control System, A Case Study in Hard Real-Time Design and Implementation,* YCS 190, Department of Computer Science, University of York, 1993.

[20]   W E Veseley, *Fault Tree Handbook*, System Safety Office, US Nuclear Regulatory Commission, 1981.

[21]   Society of Automotive Engineers, *Design Analysis Procedures for FailureModes, Effects and Criticality Analysis (FMECA)*, Aerospace Recommended Practices (ARP) 926, 1967.

[22]   S J Clarke, J A McDermid, *Software Fault Trees and Weakest Pre-conditions: A Comparison and Analysis*, Software Engineering Journal, July 1993.

[23]   N G Leveson, P R Harvey, *Software Fault Tree Analysis*, Journal of Systems and Software, 1983.

[24]   P Fenelon, J A McDermid, *An Integrated Toolset for Software Safety Analysis*, Journal of Systems and Software, July 1993.

[25]   D J Pavey, L A Winsborrow, *Demonstrating the Equivalence of Source Code and PROM Contents*, in Proceedings of the Fourth European Workshop on Dependable Computing, Prague, 1992.

[26]   British Computer Society, *Industry Structure Model*, 1992.

---

[9] This, and the other study reports are available from YSE; work is under way to make the reports available by FTP. A slightly revised version of the langugae definition is available through the University as YCS 201.

Ada: Towards Maturity
Ed. L. Collingbourne
IOS Press 1993

Automatic Proof of the Absence of Run-time Errors

Jon GARNSWORTHY, Ian O'NEILL and Bernard CARRÉ
Program Validation Ltd., 26 Queen's Terrace, Southampton, SO1 1BQ, ENGLAND

Abstract. The use of modern high-level languages and their compilers allows a large number of programming errors to be trapped at the compilation stage, through increasingly sophisticated static-semantic checks. There does remain however an important class of errors against which protection is not immediately provided – of "run-time" errors. In a safety-critical system even a well-signalled run-time error could be quite as hazardous as any other kind of malfunction.

This paper explains how the formal definition of SPARK can be used to generate systematically the theorems to establish absence of important classes of run-time errors, such as range constraint violations, and shows that many of these theorems can be proved automatically. It is pointed out that the generation and automatic proof of these theorems is facilitated by defensive programming and the inclusion through formal annotations of low-level design assumptions.

1. Introduction

For safety-critical applications the behaviour of software must be *predictable*, under all possible operating conditions. SPARK, an annotated subset of Ada, has been designed to eliminate ambiguities and insecurities of the full Ada language, and thereby to facilitate rigorous design and reasoning about Ada program behaviour [1, 2]. Its use is supported by the SPARK Examiner, a software tool which checks conformance of a program to the rules of SPARK, and performs its static code analysis, i.e. control-, data- and information-flow analysis [3]; the Examiner can also generate verification conditions, to prove that a program meets a given formal specification [2].

Compliance with the rules of SPARK, enforced by the Examiner, provides protection against many well-known kinds of programming errors (e.g. failure to initialise variables), and also more obscure defects (such as side-effects of function subprograms, and aliasing of procedure parameters), as well as the kinds of static-semantic errors that are detected by an Ada compiler. There does remain however an important class of errors against which protection is not immediately provided – that of *run-time errors*.

In this paper we consider the sources of run-time errors in Ada programs and then the practical possibilities of proving that a SPARK program will never give rise to a run-time error, i.e. that during its execution no pre-defined Ada exception will be raised.

The next section considers run-time errors in Ada programs and the importance of guaranteeing that they will not occur. The following section, because of its importance to how we construct the proof obligations for the absence of run-time errors, describes the formal definition of SPARK. We then describe how the proof obligations are derived from the formal definition and a SPARK program. The paper next considers what form these proof obligations take and whether an automatic prover will be able to prove them without manual intervention. Finally, it outlines some planned developments for tools to support the process of automatic proof of the absence of run-time errors.

Table 1: Sources of Run-Time Errors in Ada Programs

Exception	Source
CONSTRAINT_ERROR	*access check, discriminant check*, index check, *length check*, range check
NUMERIC_ERROR	division check, overflow check
PROGRAM_ERROR	*erroneous execution, incorrect order dependence, return not executed in function subprogram, elaboration check*
STORAGE_ERROR	exhaustion of dynamic heap storage, 'stack overflow'
TASKING_ERROR	*exceptions raised during intertask communication*

2. Run-time Errors

It has always been considered important to detect and report language violations, but until recently such errors have been viewed very much in terms of the practical capabilities of compilers: language errors have been classified as "compilation errors" (covering syntactic and static-semantic errors) and "run-time errors" (including for instance range violations of values of dynamically-evaluated expressions). Whilst attempts are made to detect as many errors as possible at compilation time, their detection at run-time has usually been regarded as a tolerable alternative. In a safety-critical real-time system however, even a well-signalled run-time error could be quite as hazardous as any other kind of malfunction; for our purposes *all* language violations must be detected prior to program execution.

A list of the possible kinds of run-time errors in an Ada program, with the associated exceptions, is given in Table 1. Just as Ada is richer in the language constructs it supports than a language such as Pascal, it also has more kinds of run-time errors; for example, an attempt to assign an array value to an array variable where the length of the variable differs from that of the value will give rise to a pre-defined exception in Ada, but the problem could never even arise in many simpler languages. Use before elaboration is an example of a kind of run-time error that is specific to Ada.

SPARK, as a subset of Ada with additional static semantic rules, does not allow many of these kinds of run-time errors; either the source feature has been removed (e.g. TASKING_ERROR can never be raised in a SPARK program) or the problem is detectable at "compile-time" (e.g. it is statically determinable in SPARK that a subtype indication is compatible with the type mark in a subtype definition). Those kinds of errors given in italics in the Table cannot occur in a SPARK program. The SPARK language severely reduces the possibilties for introducing the remaining ones: for example dynamic heap storage cannot be used explicitly by the programmer so this is only a source of run-time errors if the use of the dynamic heap is introduced by the compiler - and given the semantics of SPARK, the programmer can calculate the program's memory requirements prior to execution and so avoid STORAGE_ERROR entirely.

The problem to be addressed here is that of proving that none of the following checks will fail during the execution of a SPARK program: index check, range check, division check and overflow check. In the first instance, this is done by associating with each possible instance of a run-time error in a SPARK program some *proof obligation*, a theorem we must prove in order to show that the run-time error will not occur [4]. These theorems can be derived systematically using the formal definition of SPARK, as indicated below.

3. The SPARK Formal Definition

The proof obligations to show the absence of run-time errors have been obtained from the formal definition of SPARK: a mathematical definition of the well-formation rules and semantics. The form and other possible uses of the formal definition are discussed in [2]; here we only explain the derivation of the proof obligations.

3.1   Specification Language

The formal definition of SPARK has been written as a *structured operational semantics*[5] (see [6] for a more gentle introduction) and we have chosen to use Z notation [7], extended with inference rules, to express this definition. The choice of Z was driven by our desire for readability of the definition rather than the ability to execute it or prove theorems about it. Z is also widely used.

Inference rules are traditionally used in operational semantics to define both predicates and transition relations. Although we could have expressed these directly in Z we have chosen to use inference rules, both because this is accepted practice in defining an operational semantics and because they enhance the readability of the semantics.

3.2   Structured Operational Semantics

An operational semantics describes the evaluation of the program on some abstract machine: transitions in the state of this machine are defined for each stage of the evaluation (the definition therefore defines a *transition system*). In a structured operational semantics the main component of a state of this machine is a term of the abstract syntax; the structure of the definition follows from the structure of the language itself. To describe the semantics of statements, the state of the transition system includes: the environment, which contains the types of variables and the definition of procedures; the store, which contains the values of the variables; and a term from the abstract syntax. A transition is defined by a *re-write rule*. For a statement, for example, the re-write rule would take the form:

$$\varepsilon, \sigma \vdash Stmt \Rightarrow \sigma'$$

This may be read as: executing the statement *Stmt* in the environment ε transforms the store σ to the store σ', i.e. the execution of a statement changes the values of some variables.

The relationships between the transitions of the machine are expressed using inference rules. Figure 1 shows the two rules associated with the if-then-else statement. The first rule may be read as: given that the condition *cond* evaluates to *true* in the environment ε and the store σ and that execution of the if-part *ifpart* in the environment ε transforms the store σ to

$\forall \varepsilon: Env; \sigma, \sigma': Store; IfElStmt$

•

$$\frac{\varepsilon, \sigma \vdash_e cond \Rightarrow enumval\ true}{\varepsilon, \sigma \vdash ifpart \Rightarrow \sigma'}$$
$$\frac{}{\varepsilon, \sigma \vdash ifel(\theta IfElStmt) \Rightarrow \sigma'}$$

$\forall \varepsilon: Env; \sigma, \sigma': Store; IfElStmt$

•

$$\frac{\varepsilon, \sigma \vdash_e cond \Rightarrow enumval\ false}{\varepsilon, \sigma \vdash elsepart \Rightarrow \sigma'}$$
$$\frac{}{\varepsilon, \sigma \vdash ifel(\theta IfElStmt) \Rightarrow \sigma'}$$

(a)   (b)

Figure 1: The inference rules for the *if-then-else* statement

$$\forall \epsilon : Env; \sigma : Store; AsgnStmt; v : Val$$

$$|$$

$$v \in int\_tmark\_range \; \epsilon \; var$$

$$\bullet$$

$$\frac{\epsilon, \sigma \vdash_e val \Rightarrow v}{\epsilon, \sigma \vdash_s asgn(\theta AsgnStmt) \Rightarrow \sigma \oplus \{var \mapsto v\}}$$

Figure 2: The Inference rule for an integer assignment statement

the store σ', then execution of the if-then-else statement in the environment ϵ transforms the store σ to the store σ'. The second rule states what occurs when the condition evaluates to *false*.

The "meaning" of a program can be determined via the repeated application of the re-write and inference rules until some final state is reached, with the result held in the store. This approach to the formal definition accords well with our intuitive understanding of the way in which the language is executed.

3.3 Side-conditions

To control whether a transition should apply or not the inference rules are written with *side-conditions*. For example, Figure 2 shows the inference rule for an assignment statement involving integer variables. The rule is preceded by a side-condition which states that the value *v* of the expression *val* belongs to the range of the variable *var*. It is the violation of such side-conditions which determines the occurence of run-time errors.

A side-condition is traditionally placed to the right of the line in the inference rule that separates the antecedents from the conclusion, hence the name "side-condition". Since we are writing in Z however, we have chosen to place the side-condition in the more usual place for a quantified expression.

3.4 Static Semantics

Not all the terms in the abstract syntax are given a meaning by the kinds of rules shown in Figures 1 and 2. For example, in Figure 2, there are no side-conditions which express the visibility or type rules of SPARK. A separate transition system that captures the well-formation rules which are not dependent on the values which variables may take has been defined. This transition system forms the *static semantics* of SPARK. The rules captured in the static semantics are those checked by the SPARK Examiner; indeed, the formal definition of SPARK has proved very useful in our continuing development of this tool.

The final state of the transition system that defines the static semantics includes the environment and this is used by the second part of the semantics: the *dynamic semantics*.

3.5 Dynamic Semantics

The definition of the dynamic semantics is simplified by the fact that it can assume many properties of the program, e.g. that it is well-typed, and that the environment is as constructed by the static semantics. The well-formation rules that appear in the dynamic semantics are those which constrain the computed values which expressions may assume in a legal execution - which are usually only checked at run-time and whose general validity can only be established by proof methods. For programs which give rise to run-time errors the transistion system will never reach an acceptable final state: either it reaches some state from which there is no applicable transition, or it never terminates. The second of these is caused in SPARK by infinite loops; these are important but the proof of their absence is well understood [8] and so we will not consider them further here.

3.6   Overflow During Evaluation

Let us consider the assignment statement

$$c := a + b - 1$$

where a, b and c are variables declared as in Figure 3, and both a and b have the value 64. The implementation could use an eight-bit (signed) integer to represent *and evaluate* this expression and therefore overflow could occur during evaluation even though the final value was within the type; i.e. we would be able to show the side-condition of the inference rule for integer assignment was satisfied even though the statement would give rise to a run-time error: the side-condition is not strong enough in this instance. Run-time contraints on the evaluation of expressions which are implementation-dependent are not captured by the formal definition. Whether it is possible to define a set of proof obligations to show that run-time constraints of this kind are met is currently under investigation.

4. Generating the Proof Obligations

The proof obligations, to establish absence of "run-time" errors in any execution of a

```
type SmallInteger is range -128 .. 127;

procedure r (a, b: in      SmallInteger;
             c, d:      out SmallInteger)
--# derives c, d from a, b;
--# pre a in -128..127 and b in -128..127;
is
begin
  if a >= 0 and b >= 0
  then
    if a >= b
    then
      --# check a - b in -128..127;
      c := a - b;
    else
      --# check b - a in -128..127;
      c := b - a;
    end if;
  elsif a < 0 and b < 0
  then
      --# check -(b + 1) in -128..127;
      c := -(b + 1);
  else
    --# check a + b in -128..127;
    c := a + b;
  end if;
  --# check 2 /= 0 and (a + b) / 2 in -128..127;
  d := (a + b) / 2;
end r;
```

Figure 3: Code fragment

particular SPARK program, can be derived systematically from the side-conditions associated with the inference rules of the SPARK dynamic semantics. We can capture the requirement for the validity of the side-conditions and so generate theorems which show whether the proof obligations are met by inserting *check* statements into SPARK programs, as in Figure 3 for example.

4.1   Check Statements

A check statement is a SPARK annotation which expresses a constraint (a boolean expression) which the programmer wishes to claim to be *true*. Examples of check statements can be seen in Figure 3. A check statement is introduced by --# and is recognised by the SPARK Examiner; but as an Ada comment the check statement is ignored by an Ada compiler. The *verification condition generator*, which is built into the SPARK Examiner and described in [2], can then be used to generate a *verification condition* (a theorem) that shows whether the claim is *true* or not. There is, of course, a third possibility which is that we cannot show the verification condition to be either *true* or *false*; we consider this possibility in more detail later.

The language we use to write the expressions in check statements is an extended form of SPARK expressions. There are three main extensions:

1. the logical operators *implies* (->) and *is equivalent to* (<->);
2. universal and existential quantification (for example, the expression
    ```
    for all i : Index => a(i) > 0
    ```
    is true if and only if all the elements of a are greater than zero);
3. a notation for the 'updating' of composite objects (for example, the expression
    ```
    a[i => a(j); j => a(i)]
    ```
    has the value of the array a with its ith and j^{th} elements exchanged).

The insertion of the check statements which show the absence of run-time errors is currently a manual process. However, because the number of check statements required may be very large, it is planned to make the SPARK Examiner include them automatically as it generates verification conditions.

4.2   The Proof Obligations

Each verification condition consists of two parts: hypotheses and conclusions. To prove a verification condition, we assume that the hypotheses are true, and establish that the conclusions follow from them. The verification conditions associated with run-time checks usually have particularly simple conclusions – for example, that a value belongs to a range.

The hypotheses of a verification condition consist of the *traversal condition* of the execution path that terminates at the point in the code at which the check statement is located, plus the conclusions following from verification conditions earlier on the path. Thus, if an assignment is made to a variable on some path, for example, then we can assume that variable belongs to its subtype when discharging proof obligations for statements occurring subsequently on that path.   Similar reasoning is applied by compilers, in eliminating redundant run-time checks from compiled code.

As an example of the verification conditions arising from an annotated SPARK text, consider the code fragment in Figure 3. The pre-condition used here is derived from the types of the imported parameters. No post-condition is needed: checks that the exported variables are updated with values appropriate to their subtypes are placed where the updating occurs, while flow analysis ensures that all exported variables are updated. Figure

```
Verification_Condition_1.            Verification_Condition_2.
H1:    - 128 <= a.                   H1:    - 128 <= a.
H2:    a <= 127.                     H2:    a <= 127.
H3:    - 128 <= b.                   H3:    - 128 <= b.
H4:    b <= 127.                     H4:    b <= 127.
H5:    a >= 0.                       H5:    a >= 0.
H6:    b >= 0.                       H6:    b >= 0.
H7:    a >= b.                       H7:    not (a >= b).
       ->                                   ->
C1:    - 128 <= a - b.              C1:    - 128 <= b - a.
C2:    a - b <= 127.                C2:    b - a <= 127.

Verification_Condition_3.            Verification_Condition_4.
H1:    - 128 <= a.                   H1:    - 128 <= a.
H2:    a <= 127.                     H2:    a <= 127.
H3:    - 128 <= b.                   H3:    - 128 <= b.
H4:    b <= 127.                     H4:    b <= 127.
H5:    not ((a >= 0) and (b >= 0)).  H5:    not ((a >= 0) and (b >= 0)).
H6:    a < 0.                         H6:    not ((a < 0) and (b < 0)).
H7:    b < 0.                                ->
       ->                            C1:    - 128 <= a + b.
C1:    - 128 <=  - (b + 1).         C2:    a + b <= 127.
C2:    - (b + 1) <= 127.
```

Figure 4: Verification conditions from above code

4 shows a sample of the verification conditions derived from the check statements embedded in the SPARK source text: there is one for each path from the start of the procedure to a check statement. A verification condition's hypotheses are labelled H1, H2 etc., while the conclusions are labelled C1, C2 etc.: the hypotheses are implicitly conjoined (with a logical *and*), as are the conclusions, while the whole formula is a single implication, thus:

$$(H1 \wedge H2 \wedge \ldots) \Rightarrow (C1 \wedge C2 \wedge \ldots).$$

The form of presentation shown in Figure 4 is used by both the SPARK Automatic Simplifier and the SPADE Proof Checker, whose use we consider in the next section.

5. Automatic Proof

Since run-time proof obligations are associated with many of the syntactic categories of SPARK, many statements in a program will give rise to proof obligations, often a multiplicity of them. The manual proof of all these formulae would not be feasible, but since they are in large part relatively simple the process is amenable to some automation. The SPARK Automatic Simplifier, a tool for simplifying theorems, based on components from the interactive SPADE Proof Checker [9], is well suited to this task. Currently, work centres on the generation of the verification conditions in forms for which automatic proof is as easy as possible, for instance through assertion propagation, automatic strengthening of loop-invariants, extraction of invariants from exit tests and special techniques for arrays.

The Simplifier consists of a number of proof components which it employs to reduce the constituent expressions of each verification condition to a simpler form; some user control over the extent of the simplifications to be performed can be exercised via the command line. The main components of the Simplifier are:

- an expression *standardiser*, which attempts to find equivalence between expressions by converting them to a standard form (e.g. both *b+a* and *1*a-(0-b)* have the same standard form, *a+b*).

```
@@@@@@@@@@  VC: Verification_Condition_1.  @@@@@@@@@@
***  Proved C1:  - 128 <= a - b
     using hypothesis H7.
***  Proved C2:  a - b <= 127
     using hypotheses H2 & H6.
***  PROVED VC.

@@@@@@@@@@  VC: Verification_Condition_2.  @@@@@@@@@@
>>>  Restructured hypothesis H7 into:
     >>>  H7:  a < b
***  Proved C1:  - 128 <= b - a
     using hypothesis H7.
***  Proved C2:  b - a <= 127
     using hypotheses H4 & H5.
***  PROVED VC.

@@@@@@@@@@  VC: Verification_Condition_3.  @@@@@@@@@@
>>>  Restructured hypothesis H5 into:
     >>>  H5:  a < 0 or b < 0
***  Proved C1:  - 128 <= - (b + 1)
     via its standard form, which is:
     Std.Fm C1:  - b > - 128
     using hypothesis H4.
***  Proved C2:  - (b + 1) <= 127
     via its standard form, which is:
     Std.Fm C2:  b > - 129
     using hypothesis H3.
***  PROVED VC.

@@@@@@@@@@  VC: Verification_Condition_4.  @@@@@@@@@@
>>>  Restructured hypothesis H5 into:
     >>>  H5:  a < 0 or b < 0
>>>  Restructured hypothesis H6 into:
     >>>  H6:  0 <= a or 0 <= b
```

Figure 5: Simplification log for above formulae

- a *simplifier* with specific rules for the data types of SPARK, e.g. rules to simplify expressions involving array elements and updates, and record field accesses.
- an *inference engine* which attempts to infer the conclusions from the hypotheses, using various rules (e.g. to infer $a>b$, try finding a c such that both $a > c$ and $c \geq b$ hold).
- a *contradiction-hunter*, which attempts to establish a contradiction between hypotheses as a way of discharging a verification condition.

The SPARK Automatic Simplifier generates both a simplified set of verification conditions and a log of the simplifications and inferences which it performed on each verification condition. For the verification conditions shown in Figure 4, for instance, the simplifier produces a log describing its actions as shown in Figure 5 and the simplified verification conditions shown in Figure 6. It will be seen that the fourth verification condition is not proved automatically. In fact, it is provable but the Simplifier is not sufficiently powerful: the proof requires case analysis on the two disjunctions (H5 and H6), which the Simplifier does not perform.

The SPADE Proof Checker can be used interactively to construct proofs that the Simplifier cannot carry out, if they are in fact provable. For the fourth verification condition in the above example, for instance, the Proof Checker was used to carry out the proof by cases that the Simplifier is unable to perform.

```
Verification_Condition_1.
*** true .              /* all conclusions proved */

Verification_Condition_2.
*** true .              /* all conclusions proved */

Verification_Condition_3.
*** true .              /* all conclusions proved */

Verification_Condition_4.
H1:    - 128 <= a .
H2:    a <= 127 .
H3:    - 128 <= b .
H4:    b < = 127 .
H5:    a < 0 or b < 0 .
H6:    0 <= a or 0 <= b .
       ->
C1:    - 128 <= a + b .
```

Figure 6: Simplified verification conditions

6. An Example

The following example illustrates the application of the concepts and techniques described above.

6.1   The Package Stacks

Figure 7 shows the package specification for an abstract data type representing integer stacks of a fixed maximum size; Figure 8 shows an implementation of its procedure Push. If

```
package Stacks
is
    type Stack is private;

    function Empty (s : Stack) return boolean;

    function Full (s : Stack) return boolean;

    procedure Push (s : in out Stack;
                    x : in      Integer);
    --# derives s from s, x;

    procedure Pop (s : in out Stack;
                   x :     out Integer);
    --# derives s, x from s;

private
    MaxDepth : constant Integer := 100;
    subtype StackPointer is Integer range 0..MaxDepth;
    subtype StackIndex is Integer range 1..MaxDepth;
    type StackContent is array (StackIndex) of Integer;
    type Stack is record
                    Pointer : StackPointer;
                    Content : StackContent;
                  end record;
end Stacks;
```

Figure 7

```
procedure Push (s : in out Stack;
                x : in      Integer)
is
begin
  s.Pointer := s.Pointer + 1;
  s.Content(s.Pointer) := x;
end Push
```

Figure 8

we annotate the procedure with check statements (as shown in Figure 9) and then use the SPARK Examiner to generate the verification conditions we obtain the theorems of Figure 10. The hypotheses of the first of these verification conditions follow from the type of the field pointer of the variable s. (In the logic in which the verification conditions are given, field accesses are represented by function application.) In the second verification condition the first two hypotheses are indentical to those in the first verification condition; the other two hypotheses carry forward the conclusions of the first verification condition.

The second verification condition is proved automatically by the Simplifier (in the same way, we would expect a compiler to eliminate an index check for that array access) but the first one cannot be proved: the code has been written with the unstated assumption that the procedure Push will not be called if the stack is full.

With SPARK, we can add this assumption to our program by stating it as a pre-condition of the procedure Push, as in Figure 11. In order to allow us to prove the verification conditions we also have to extend the declaration of the function Full with some additional information, as shown in Figure 12. It will be noted that here the specification of the value returned by the function Full is identical to its implementation; of course, this is not always the case.

```
procedure Push (s : in out Stack;
                x : in      Integer)
is
begin
  --# check s.Pointer + 1 in StackPointer;
  s.Pointer := s.Pointer + 1;
  --# check s.Pointer in StackIndex;
  s.Content(s.Pointer) := x;
end Push;
```

Figure 9

```
Verification_Condition_1.
H1:     0 <= fld_pointer(s).
H2:     fld_pointer(s) <= 100.
        ->
C1:     0 <= fld_pointer(s) + 1.
C2      fld_pointer(s) + 1 <= 100.

Verification_Condition_2.
H1:     0 <= fld_pointer(s).
H2:     fld_pointer(s) <= 100.
H3:     0 <= fld_pointer(s) + 1.
H4:     fld_pointer(s) + 1 <= 100.
        ->
C1:     1 <= fld_pointer(upf_pointer(s, fld_pointer(s) + 1)).
C2:     fld_pointer(upf_pointer(s, fld_pointer(s) + 1)) <= 100.
```

Figure 10

```
function Full (s : Stack) return boolean
--# return s.Pointer = MaxDepth;
is
begin
   return s.Pointer = MaxDepth;
end Full;
```

Figure 11

```
procedure Push (s : in out Stack;
                x : in      Integer);
--# derives s from s, x;
--# pre not Full(s);
```

Figure 12

The verification conditions for the procedure `Push` after inclusion of its pre-condition are shown in Figure 13. It is not currently possible for the Simplifier to discharge the first of the two verification conditions because it does not yet have access to the definition of the function `Full` at this point; at present we must use the SPADE Proof Checker.

By a similar argument we can prove the absence of run-time errors in the procedure `Pop` by introducing a pre-condition of

```
not Empty(s)
```

SPARK requires that we give dependency annotations (`derives...`) specifying the information-flow associated with a procedure: these are specifications, but weak ones. The addition of pre-conditions, such as those we have given to the procedures `Push` and `Pop`, make the specification stronger, but we are still not supplying a full formal specification of the package `Stacks`.

6.2   The Procedure `Negate`

We will now employ the package `Stacks` in a simple calculator. First let us consider an operation to negate the topmost integer in a stack; an annotated implementation of this is shown in Figure 14. To simplify our discussion, when annotating this procedure we have chosen to ignore the fact that the expression `-x` may give rise to a run-time error, for example if `x = Integer'FIRST`.

```
Verification_Condition_1.
H1:     not full(s).
H2:     0 <= fld_pointer(s).
H3:     fld_pointer(s) <= 100.
        ->
C1:     0 <= fld_pointer(s) + 1.
C2      fld_pointer(s) + 1 <= 100.

Verification_Condition_2.
H1:     not full(s).
H2:     0 <= fld_pointer(s).
H3:     fld_pointer(s) <= 100.
H4:     0 <= fld_pointer(s) + 1.
H5:     fld_pointer(s) + 1 <= 100.
        ->
C1:     1 <= fld_pointer(upf_pointer(s, fld_pointer(s) + 1)).
C2:     fld_pointer(upf_pointer(s, fld_pointer(s) + 1)) <= 100.
```

Figure 13

The verification condition associated with the first check statement is shown in Figure 15. Clearly we cannot prove it to be true; indeed, we cannot infer from the text of the procedure Negate, that its execution will not result in a call of the procedure Pop when the stack s is empty. There are two ways of overcoming this problem.

The first solution is to add a pre-condition to the declaration of the procedure Negate, prohibiting its execution if the stack is empty (see Figure 16). Of course, inclusion of this pre-condition introduces proof obligations – in the calling environment – to ensure that wherever the procedure is called the pre-condition does hold. The resulting verification condition is shown in Figure 17 and can be immediately discharged by the Simplifier.

An alternative approach is to use "defensive programming" - introducing a conditional statement into the body of the procedure Negate, as in Figure 18, so that the procedure Pop is not called when the stack s is empty. The resulting verification conditions are identical to those generated in the first approach (see Figure 17). The body of the procedure Negate, shown in Figure 18, leaves open the question of what action should be taken if the stack is found to be empty.

Let us now consider the validity of the check condition associated with the call to the procedure Push. We could again use a conditional statement as was suggested in connection with the call of the procedure Pop. However, whereas it is reasonable to include such a check before the call of procedure Pop, to confirm that the stack is not full immediately after we have popped a value from it must be unreasonable - the stack *cannot* be full immediately after a call to the procedure Pop. How can we record this claim? We extend our weak specification of the procedure Pop slightly by giving a post-condition for it, as in Figure 19. This post-condition will give rise to a proof obligation, associated with

```
procedure Negate
--# global   s;
--# derives s from s;
is
   x : Integer;
begin
   --# check not Stacks.Empty(s);
   Stacks.Pop(s, x);
   --# check not Stacks.Full(s);
   Stacks.Push(s, -x);
end Negate;
```

Figure 14

```
Verification_Condition_1.
H1:     true.
        ->
C1:     not stacks__empty(s).
```

Figure 15

```
procedure Negate
--# global   s;
--# derives s from s;
--# pre not Stacks.Empty(s);
```

Figure 16

```
Verification_Condition_1.
H1:     not stacks__empty(s).
        ->
C1:     not stacks__empty(s).
```

Figure 17

```
if not Stacks.Empty(s)
then
   --# check not Stacks.Empty(s);
   Stacks.Pop(s, x);
   --# check not Stacks.Full(s);
   Stacks.Push(s, -x);
else
   null; -- Error action
end if;
```

Figure 18

```
procedure Pop( s : in out Stack;
               x :     out Integer)
--# derives s, x from s;
--# pre   not Empty(s);
--# post not Full(s);
```

Figure 19

the body of the procedure Pop, to show that this claim is true; but this claim will be assumed automatically immediately following any call to the procedure Pop.

It is important to note that we are still not providing a full formal specification of the procedure Pop; we are capturing our design assumptions within the text of the program in a form that is both familiar to the programmer and mechanically checkable.

6.3　The Procedure Add

To show how this process can be pursued further – still without producing a formal specification, but continuing to capture design assumptions in greater and greater detail – we will now consider a procedure to add the two topmost numbers of the stack s together.

It is obvious that for a procedure which adds two numbers we require the stack to have a depth of at least two. We may not want to make the depth of the Stack available within the executable code but we can still make it available for use in the annotations. We do this by adding to the specification of the stack a *proof function* Depth, as shown in Figure 20. A proof function is a function that is only visible in annotations; it cannot have a body. The proof function Depth can then be used to construct weak specifications of other subprograms. For example Figure 21 shows a new specification for the procedure Pop, stating that it may only be called with a stack that has a depth of at least 1; after it has been called the depth of the stack will have decreased by 1 and the depth of the stack will be less

```
--# function Depth (s : Stack) return Integer;
```

Figure 20

```
procedure Pop (s : in out Stack;
               x :     out Integer);
--# derives s, x from s;
--# pre   Depth(s) >= 1;
--# post Depth(s) = Depth(s~) - 1 and
--#      Depth(s) < MaxDepth;
```

Figure 21

```
--# function Depth (s : Stack) return Integer;
--# return s.Pointer;
```

Figure 22

```
procedure Add
--# global  s;
--# derives s from s;
--# pre Stacks.Depth(s) >= 2;
is
begin
   --# check Stacks.Depth(s) >= 1;
   Stacks.Pop(s, x);
   --# check Stacks.Depth(s) >= 1;
   Stacks.Pop(s, y);
   --# check Stacks.Depth(s) < MaxDepth;
   Stacks.Push(s, x + y);
end Add;
```

Figure 23

```
Verification_Condition_1
H1:      stacks__depth(s) >= 2.
         ->
C1:      stacks__depth(s) >= 1.

Verification_Condition_2.
H1:      stacks__depth(s) >= 2.
H2:      stacks__depth(s) >= 1.
H3:      stacks__depth(s__1) = stack_depth(s) - 1.
H4:      stacks__depth(s__1) < stacks__maxdepth.
         ->
C1       stacks__depth(s__1) >= 1.

Verification_Condition_3.
H1:      stacks__depth(s) >= 2.
H2:      stacks__depth(s) >= 1.
H3:      stacks__depth(s__1) = stacks__depth(s) - 1.
H4:      stacks__depth(s__1) < stacks__maxdepth.
H5:      stacks__depth(s__1) >= 1.
H6:      stacks__depth(s__2) = stack_depth(s__1) - 1.
H7:      stacks__depth(s__2) < stacks__maxdepth.
         ->
C1:      stacks__depth(s__2) < stacks__maxdepth.
```

Figure 24

than MaxDepth. This last conjunct is derived from the invariant of the stack type; SPARK does not (yet) provide a mechanism to state the invariant directly so we have to add this conjunct to the post-condition explicitly. (The tilde ~ in a post-condition indicates the initial value of a variable.) Similarly, we can specify the procedure Push. Although the proof function Depth has no body it will require a definition; we give this in the body of the package Stacks (see Figure 22). In addition, we place the constant MaxDepth in the package specification of Stacks.

Figure 23 shows the declaration of the procedure Add annotated with a suitable pre-condition and check statements; the verification conditions are shown in Figure 24. Note that we have again ignored the possibility of the failure of a range check associated with the expression x + y. The value of the stack on entry to the procedure Add is denoted by s, and s__1 and s__2 denote its value after the first and second calls respectively of the procedure Pop.

7. Conclusions

The work reported here has demonstrated that, employing the formal definition of SPARK, it is possible to generate systematically the theorems to establish absence of important classes of run-time errors, such as range constraint violations. Many of these theorems have very simple conclusions (for instance, that a value belongs to a range) and a large proportion of them can be proved automatically. Work is now in hand further to mechanise these processes, through

- extension of the SPARK Examiner, to mechanise entirely the generation of proof obligations to establish absence of such errors, with the theorems being documented to allow readers to relate them easily to the source code, and
- inclusion in the SPARK Automatic Simplifier of more powerful simplification strategies, tuned specifically to proving typical run-time check conditions, and a facility for consulting rule files specific to an application.

With these in place it will become much easier to address pragmatic issues, such as how to organise assertion propagation and other devices for strengthening hypotheses, so that theorems are produced in forms for which automatic proof is as simple as possible.

Topics on which further work is required are overflow during expression evaluation, and real arithmetic in SPARK (which remains to be treated in the formal definition).

As has been illustrated, the reasoning process in proving the absence of run-time errors in a program may reveal to the programmer potentially hazardous features of which he was not aware. The proposed facilities, encouraging this kind of exploration, should help in producing well-designed and formally-documented code, in which it is clear that the potential for run-time errors has been properly addressed.

8. Acknowledgements

The development of the Examiner and the formal definition has been supported by contracts from DRA Farnborough and DRA Malvern respectively; in particular, the work on run-time errors reported in this paper was partially funded by DRA Farnborough.

References

[1] B.A. Carré, T.J. Jennings, F.J. Maclennan, P.F. Farrow and J.R. Garnsworthy, SPARK - the SPADE Ada Kernel (Edition 3.1), 1992. *Obtainable from Program Validation Ltd.*

[2] B.A. Carré, J.R. Garnsworthy and D.W.R. Marsh, SPARK: A Safety-Related Ada Subset. In W.J. Taylor (Ed.), Ada in Transition. ISBN 90 5199 133 4. IOS Press, Amsterdam, 1992, pp. 31 - 45.

[3] J. Bergeretti and B.A. Carré, Information-Flow and Data-Flow Analysis of **while**-Programs. ACM Transactions on Programming Languages and Systems, Vol. 7, No. 1, January 1985, pp. 37-61.

[4] S.M. German, Automating proof of the absence of common run-time errors. In Proceedings 5th ACM Conference on Principles of Programming Languages. ACM, New York., 1978.

[5] G.D. Plotkin, A Structural Approach to Operational Semantics. Report: DAIMI FN-19, Computer Science Department, Aarhus University, Denmark. September 1981.

[6] H.R. Nielson and F. Nielson, Semantics with Applications, A Formal Introduction. ISBN 0 471 92980. Wiley, 1992.

[7] J.M. Spivey, The Z Notation: a reference manual, second edition. ISBN 0 13 978529 9. Prentice-Hall, 1992.

[8] D. Gries, Science of Programming. ISBN 0 387 90641. Springer-Verlag, 1981.

[9] I.M. O'Neill, Logic Programming Tools and Techniques for Imperative Program Verification. Ph.D. Thesis, University of Southampton Department of Electronics and Computer Science, April 1987.

Ada: Towards Maturity
Ed. L. Collingbourne
IOS Press 1993

A Formal Design Method
for Real-Time Ada Software

Michael G. Hinchey

University of Cambridge Computer Laboratory
New Museums Site, Pembroke Street, Cambridge CB2 3QG, UK

and

Digital Equipment Corporation Systems Research Center
130 Lytton Avenue, Palo Alto, CA 95401, USA

Abstract. A formal design method, based on an extended version of Receptive Process Theory, which is suitable for use in the design of real-time systems is described. The method is particularly appropriate for use with Ada software, as it can fully exploit Ada's advanced features such as tasking, multiple entry-points, exception handling, etc., and also supports asynchronous communication.

1. Introduction

Mathematical Science shows what <u>is</u>. It is the language of unseen relations between things. But to use & apply that language we must be able fully to appreciate, to feel, to seize, the unseen, the unconscious. Imagination too shows what <u>is</u>, the <u>is</u> that is beyond the senses. Hence she is or should be especially cultivated by the truly Scientific, – those who which to enter into the worlds around us!

Augusta Ada Lovelace, essay written 5th January 1841

Failures of complex real-time and safety-critical systems — the very classes of system for which Ada is so appropriate — have received increased media attention in recent years, and have caused concern amongst the general public and the developers of such systems alike.

It is now widely acccepted that informal and semi-formal methods are not suitable for use in the specification and design of complex systems. Such systems require more formal approaches, whereby correctness issues can be addressed and anticipated behaviour can be verified [1]. But, the strengths of most design methods used in practice lie in the graphical and semi-formal description of data and control flow, and of data and process structures. While they offer a means of discussing structural decomposition and the consistency of the design, correctness issues cannot be addressed in a stepwise manner as semantics are only assigned at the level of executable code [2].

The current trend is towards so-called formal methods, and there is a large body of evidence to suggest that their use can result in decreased costs and improved complexity control, while simultaneously ensuring an increase in the quality of the deliverable [3]. This trend seems certain to continue, particularly where Ada is used as the implementation language, as both the US Department of Defense and the British Ministry of Defence plan to make the use of formal methods manditory in particular applications [4, 5].

Unfortunately, while Ada has indeed been used successfully with various formal methods, none of the existing methods are designed to exploit those features of Ada that give it advantages over other programming languages – in short those features that make it a "system development" language rather than merely another programming language.

While using such methods is certainly a great improvement over traditional (structured) or *ad hoc* design methods, the advantages of using a language such as Ada are lost. No support for Ada's advanced features is available, so these must be integrated in an informal manner, increasing the risk of incorrect system behaviour.

The ideal formal design method for Ada software would provide full support for Ada's advanced features — tasking, multiple-entry points, exception handling, genericity (and other support for software reuse), etc. — and at the same time provide for the development of provably correct systems, in particular real-time systems.

Such a design method now exists — an extended version of Receptive Process Theory [6].

2. Receptive Process Theory

Receptive Process Theory (RPT) [6] represents a reworking of Hoare's language of Communicating Sequential Processes (CSP) [7, 8] under the assumption that processes are receptive.

Originally devised for use in the design of delay-insensitive circuits and broadcast networks, a very interesting discovery is that with some minor extensions RPT can be used equally effectively in the specification and design of certain classes of (distributed) real-time systems [9].

Like CSP, Receptive Process Theory is a notation for the analysis of communication patterns of cooperating programs or objects. Its language of programs, or *processes*, may be used to provide algorithmic descriptions of system behaviours, and the associated semantic model may be used to reason about system properties.

The language supports high levels of abstraction in the specification of complex systems. Unlike some other approaches to real-time Ada design [10] which require that the underlying hardware is considered at the design stage, the RPT approach takes a high-level view of the system, ignoring environmental constraints (number of available processors and their distribution, etc.) at the outset. The universe of discourse is merely viewed as consisting of a (usually large) number of sequential processes executing concurrently, which may be in communication with each other over uni-directional channels.

Even the most simple (open) system consists of a minimum of two processes — the system under consideration, and the environment in which it is executing, and with which it is in communication.

2.1. Receptive Processes

In RPT each process is assumed to be receptive, as defined by Dill [11].

A Receptive Process models the interaction between a system and its environment by input events and output events. As in CSP, the degree of granularity or abstraction is determined by the set of events that the process may engage in, i.e. its alphabet.

Just as each Receptive Process can never refuse input, the entire system (being a collection of such processes) can never block input from its environment; it must always accept input, even if this will result in undefined subsequent behaviour. Similarly, the environment is assumed to be a Receptive Process, and therefore cannot refuse input from the system. In this way, a system can never be blocked on output.

The communication primitive is therefore asynchronous. This is generally the form of communication we will want to represent in real-time systems, but at the design stage it can present another great advantage: synchronous communication as a primitive can lead to over-specification and unnecessarily exclude reasonable implementations. Conversely, asynchronous communication provides implementation freedom at little extra cost [12].

While Ada 83 does not provide support for asynchronous communication *per se*, if Ada 9X is to be suitable for use with real-time systems then explicit support for a suitable asynchronous communication mechanism will be required. RPT does not only support asynchronous communication however — synchronous communication can be modelled through the hand-shaking of processes, and hence RPT represents a very generalised reactive model of computation.

3. Process Algebra

The syntax of (extended) Receptive Process Theory is very similar to that of CSP. The notations look so similar that one could easily confuse an RPT specification with CSP. The difference is in the underlying semantics, which require quite a different interpretation.

As in CSP, a process is defined in the form:

$$event \rightarrow Process.$$

Unlike CSP, however, the only events that are of concern to us in Receptive Process Theory are communication events. However, communication events are merely special cases of events, and engagement in non-communication events can therefore be denoted by the transmission of the same message on both the input and output channels of the process. Therefore, it is more correct to say that a process is defined in the form:

$$channel?message \rightarrow Process,$$

or

$$channel!message \rightarrow Process,$$

where ? and ! denote input and output respectively.

As mentioned above, the level of abstraction of a process definition is determined by the alphabet of events. The alphabet also has an important role when it comes to applying RPT's algebraic laws to combine processes executing in parallel. It is important therefore that we specify the alphabets of each process at the outset. In RPT we must specify both the input alphabet of each process P, written iP, and its output alphabet, written oP.

These alphabets must be disjoint, the input alphabet describes the set of messages that a process may receive from its environment as input. Similarly the output alphabet describes the set of messages that it may output to its environment; the output alphabet must be non-empty or the process will be in an undesirable state, and must be modelled as $\perp$ or *Chaos*, a process that can do, or fail to do, anything.

How then can we denote the participation of a process in non-communication events by transmitting the same message on both the input and output channels? Surely this violates the requirement that the input and output alphabets are disjoint? No, in fact this is perfectly legitimate: inputting message m on channel in (denoted $in?m$) is the event $in.m$, whereas outputting message m on channel out (denoted $out!m$) is the event $out.m$. Clearly these are not the same event, and since no process can input and output on the same channel (recall that channels are uni-directional) this will never be a problem.

Process definitions can be generalised to any number of events, so it is perfectly legitimate to write process definitions in the form:

$$P = (c?m_1 \rightarrow c?m_2 \rightarrow \ldots \rightarrow c?m_n \rightarrow Q),$$

where c is a channel along which process P may input messages $m_1, \ldots, m_n$, and where

$$\mathbf{i}P = \mathbf{i}Q = \{c.m_i \mid 1 \leq i \leq n\}, \text{ and } \mathbf{o}P = \mathbf{o}Q.$$

This is not very advisable though, as when we introduce multiple channels, we must describe the behaviour of the process for each channel and each message it can carry. As a result, complex process definitions quickly become too complicated, and too large, to fit on a printed page. The former sytle is therefore preferred, although this does mean a greater number of definitions to contend with.

example 1

$\mathbf{i}P = \{in.n \mid n \in \mathcal{N}\} \cup \mathbf{i}Q$
$\mathbf{o}P = \mathbf{o}Q$
$P = (in?x \rightarrow Q)$

P is a process that eventually inputs a natural number x on its input channel in and then behaves as process Q (defined elsewhere). The process definition is said to be *input guarded*.

3.1. Choice

Obviously, processes that perform only one function are very limited. For this reason, we introduce the choice operator which allows us to define processes that can perform a number of functions.

example 2

$\mathbf{i}P = \{in.n \mid n \in \mathcal{N}\} = \mathbf{i}Q$
$\mathbf{o}P = \{out.n \mid n \in \mathcal{N}\} = \mathbf{o}Q$
$P = P_{v_0}, \text{ for some initial value } v_0 \in \mathcal{N}$
$P_v = (in?x \rightarrow Q_x)$
$Q_v = (out!v \rightarrow P_v$
$\qquad \mid in?x \rightarrow Q_x)$

In this example, P is a process that begins with a stored initial value, a natural number, and which will eventually input a new value on its input channel in. Once it records a new value it will output it on channel out, and then behaves recursively as P, unless it earlier receives input of another natural number x along channel in, in which case it will store the new value x overwriting the previously stored value. Process Q is said to be guarded with *output-guarded choice*. Later we will see a third, and final, type of guard.

The subscript in the above definition is used to record local data. We could just as easily have used a superscript, as in P^v, or parentheses, as in $P(v)$ — it is simply a matter of taste.

Notice, however, that in RPT there is no global data; instead all data in encapsulated in the process definition, in the same way that data in Ada programs is encapsulated in packages.

Choice generalises and therefore we can define processes that have any number of possible behaviours. More importantly, however, *choice* enables us to discharge our obligation of defining the behaviour of a process for each of its channels and each message that the channel can carry.

example 3

Suppose that P' is a process similar in function to process P in example 2 above, except that it may also input natural numbers on each of channels $c_1, \ldots, c_m$, but does not record these values nor output them on channel out. Although we are not going to keep a record of the input, we must define the behaviour of each channel. Thus:

$$\mathbf{i}P' = \mathbf{i}P \cup \{c_i.n \mid n \in \mathcal{N} \wedge 1 \le i \le m\} = \mathbf{i}Q$$
$$\mathbf{o}P' = \mathbf{o}P = \mathbf{o}Q$$

$P' = P'_{v_0}$, for some initial value $v_0 \in \mathcal{N}$

$$
\begin{aligned}
P'_v = (\;&in?x \rightarrow Q'_x \\
&| \; c_1?x_1 \rightarrow P'_v \\
&| \; c_2?x_2 \rightarrow P'_v \\
&\vdots \\
&| \; c_{n-1}?x_{n-1} \rightarrow P'_v \\
&| \; c_n?x_n \rightarrow P'_v\;)
\end{aligned}
$$

$$
\begin{aligned}
Q'_v = (\;&out!v \rightarrow P'_v \\
&| \; in?x \rightarrow Q'_x \\
&| \; c_1?x_1 \rightarrow Q'_v \\
&| \; c_2?x_2 \rightarrow Q'_v \\
&\vdots \\
&| \; c_{n-1}?x_{n-1} \rightarrow Q'_v \\
&| \; c_n?x_n \rightarrow Q'_v\;)
\end{aligned}
$$

The above definitions might look quite verbose, but they ensure that at every event we have defined every possible behaviour of the process.

example 4

Suppose now that we want the value stored to be reset to v_0 whenever 0 is received on channels $c_1, \ldots, c_{n-1}$, but every other value to be ignored, and that also we want to prohibit any input on channel c_n. Recall that we must define the behaviour for each input channel, so we cannot merely ignore inputs on channel c_n in our definition – we must explicitly declare such an input as undefined or $\bot$. The definition of P' is now given as:

$$\mathbf{i}P' = \mathbf{i}P \cup \{c_i.n \mid n \in \mathcal{N} \wedge 1 \le i \le m\} = \mathbf{i}Q$$
$$\mathbf{o}P' = \mathbf{o}P = \mathbf{o}Q$$

$P' = P'_{v_0}$, for some initial value $v_0 \in \mathcal{N}$

$$P'_v = (in?x \rightarrow Q'_x$$
$$| c_1?x_1 \rightarrow (P'_{v_0} \text{ if } x_1 = 0 \text{ else } P'_v)$$
$$| c_2?x_2 \rightarrow (P'_{v_0} \text{ if } x_2 = 0 \text{ else } P'_v)$$
$$\vdots$$
$$| c_{n-1}?x_{n-1} \rightarrow (P'_{v_0} \text{ if } x_{n-1} = 0 \text{ else } P'_v)$$
$$| c_n?x_n \rightarrow \perp)$$

$$Q'_v = (out!v \rightarrow P'_v$$
$$| in?x \rightarrow Q'_x$$
$$| c_1?x_1 \rightarrow (Q'_{v_0} \text{ if } x_1 = 0 \text{ else } Q'_v)$$
$$| c_2?x_2 \rightarrow (Q'_{v_0} \text{ if } x_2 = 0 \text{ else } Q'_v)$$
$$\vdots$$
$$| c_{n-1}?x_{n-1} \rightarrow (Q'_{v_0} \text{ if } x_{n-1} = 0 \text{ else } Q'_v)$$
$$| c_n?x_n \rightarrow \perp)$$

3.2. Nondeterminism

Nondeterminism in a programming language is clearly unacceptable. However, at the earlier stages of development, nondeterminism aids in maintaining higher levels of abstraction and increases the number of acceptable implementations.

Refinement can then be viewed as the systematic elimination of nondeterminism or ambiguity from the system design [13].

A nondeterministic choice operator is included in the RPT process algebra, such that the process $P = Q1 \sqcap Q2$ can behave nondeterministically as process $Q1$ or process $Q2$; we have no way of telling *a priori* which of the behaviour patterns will be chosen.

Because nondeterministic choice is both associative and commutative, it follows that it generalises to any number of operands. A restriction is, however, that all the processes in the expression much have the same alphabets, and a nondeterministic choice than can choose $\perp$ is already equivalent to $Chaos$. Thus:

$$\mathbf{i}P = \mathbf{i}Q1 \sqcap Q2 = \mathbf{i}Q1 = \mathbf{i}Q2$$
$$\mathbf{o}P = \mathbf{o}Q1 \sqcap Q2 = \mathbf{o}Q1 = \mathbf{o}Q2$$
$$P \sqcap \perp = (Q1 \sqcap Q2) \sqcap \perp = \perp$$

3.3. Parallel Composition

Simple definitions such as those given above are not very useful for describing complex systems unless we can combine them together in some way.

In RPT, we describe systems at high levels of abstraction, and assume high levels of concurrency with an infinite number of processors. We can now construct descriptions of more complex systems by placing existing definitions running in parallel, with communication between executing processes along named channels as before.

As in CSP, processes running in parallel may execute non-common events independently, but must synchronize on common events. Since events in RPT all involve communication, it follows that when one processes outputs on a given channel, and another inputs from that same channel, the two processes must synchronize on that communication event in an explicit Ada-like *rendezvous* mechanism. Other events that these two processes engage in independently of each other may be interleaved.

example 5

Suppose that processes $Q1_y$ and $Q2_w$ are defined as shown below, with the obvious input and output alphabets:

$$Q1_y = (out1!y \rightarrow Q1_y$$
$$| \ a?x \rightarrow Q1_x$$
$$| \ error?mess \rightarrow SHUTDOWN)$$
$$Q2_w = (out2!w \rightarrow Q2_w$$
$$| \ b?x \rightarrow Q2_x)$$

Then the parallel composition of $Q1_y \parallel Q2_w$ is given as:

$$Q1_y \parallel Q2_w = (out1!y \rightarrow Q1_y \parallel Q2_w$$
$$| \ a?x \rightarrow Q1_x \parallel Q2_w$$
$$| \ b?x \rightarrow Q1_y \parallel Q2_x$$
$$| \ error?mess \rightarrow (SHUTDOWN \parallel Q2_w))$$
$$\sqcap$$
$$(out2!w \rightarrow Q1_y \parallel Q2_w$$
$$| \ a?x \rightarrow Q1_x \parallel Q2_w$$
$$| \ b?x \rightarrow Q1_y \parallel Q2_x$$
$$| \ error?mess \rightarrow (SHUTDOWN \parallel Q2_w))$$

In simple English, the combined process can arbitrarily engage in either of the output events first and then behave recursively as the parallel composition. Regardless of which output event it engages in first, we must allow for the possible occurance of all of the input events before the output event has taken place; hence the duplication in the definition.

Parallel composition is more interesting, however, when one of the processes outputs on a particular channel, and the other process inputs from that channel.

example 6

$$Q1_y = (out!y \rightarrow Q1_y$$
$$| \ error?mess \rightarrow SHUTDOWN)$$
$$Q2_w = (out?x \rightarrow Q2_x)$$

Then the parallel composition of $Q1_y \parallel Q2_w$ is given as:

$$Q1_y \parallel Q2_w = (out!y \rightarrow Q1_y \parallel Q2_y$$
$$| \ error?mess \rightarrow (SHUTDOWN \parallel Q2_w))$$

That is, the parallel composition of an output event and its corresponding input event is reduced to a single output event, with the substitution of variables — note how $Q2_w$ has accepted the output value y and this has been substituted for x in the resulting composition.

3.4. Concealment

When we place a number of processes running in parallel, we actually want them to appear as a single process.

However, the fact that communication between them on common channels is still visible (as in example 6 above) makes it obvious that the processes are not fully integrated. We can overcome this by hiding or *concealing* common channels when we combine processes together.

The process $P\backslash C$ behaves like P, except that outputs in $C \subset \mathbf{o}P$ are concealed from its environment. Thus $\mathbf{i}(P\backslash C) = \mathbf{i}P$, and $\mathbf{o}(P\backslash C) = (\mathbf{o}P)\backslash C$.

The following law is required if concealment is to be eliminated from process expressions:

If $P = (!c \rightarrow P' \mid ?x \rightarrow P_x)$, then

$$P\backslash C = (skip \rightarrow (P'\backslash C) \mid ?x \rightarrow (P_x\backslash C)), \text{ if } c \in C$$

$$P\backslash C = (!c \rightarrow (P'\backslash C) \mid ?x \rightarrow (P_x\backslash C)), \text{ if } c \notin C.$$

This motivates the introduction of skip-guarded choice as a stepping-stone to the elimination of the concealment operator from finite processes. Skip-guarded choice then obeys the law that:

$$(skip \rightarrow \perp \mid ?x \rightarrow Q_x) = \perp.$$

Thus, we can make the composition of $Q1_y$ and $Q2_w$ in the last example transparent by hiding the common channel out:

example 7

$$
\begin{aligned}
Q1_y \parallel Q2_w \backslash \{out.x \mid out.x \in \mathbf{o}Q1_y\} &= (out!y \rightarrow Q1_y \parallel Q2_y \\
&\quad \mid error?mess \rightarrow (SHUTDOWN \parallel Q2_w)) \\
&\quad \backslash \{out.x \mid out.x \in \mathbf{o}Q1_y\} \\
&= (skip \rightarrow (Q1_y \parallel Q2_y)\backslash\{out.x \mid out.x \in \mathbf{o}Q1_y\} \\
&\quad \mid error?mess \rightarrow (SHUTDOWN \parallel Q2_w) \\
&\quad \backslash\{out.x \mid out.x \in \mathbf{o}Q1_y\})
\end{aligned}
$$

3.5. Labelling

The CSP labelling operator enables us to distinguish between different instances of a process definition.

Suppose for example that we wish to have two very simple processes, like process P in example 1, running in parallel, and both inputting from different channels, and with no communication between the two processes. The labelling operator enables us to achieve this; the process $i : P$ engages in the event $i.e$ everytime process P engages in event e.

example 8

With P as defined in example 1, $i : P$ is defined as:

$$i : P = (i.in?x \rightarrow i : Q)$$

So we may put two instances of process P running in parallel, communicating on the distinct channels $i.in$ and $j.in$, and with no communication between them, by defining the system as $i : P \parallel j : P$.

3.6. Change of Symbol

The final operator we describe is the change of symbol operator f, where f is a total function from the events that a process may engage in, to the new names of these events. This enables us to reuse old process definitions by changing event names to those that more accurately reflect the current problem. It can also help in overcoming the problems of having multiple instances communicating over different channels.

example 9

We now define the same simple system as in example 8, but using the change of symbol operator instead. We define functions f and g such that $f(in) = i.in$ and $g(in) = j.in$, and we assume that f and g have been defined for each of the events in the lifetime of process Q also.

The system is then given as:

$$f(P) \parallel g(P)$$
$$= f(in?x \to Q) \parallel g(in?x \to Q)$$
$$= (i.in?x \to f(Q)) \parallel (j.in?x \to g(Q))$$
$$= (i.in?x \to f(Q) \parallel g(P)) \sqcap (j.in?x \to f(P) \parallel g(Q))$$

3.7. Semantics

The further we analyse the manner in which such an engine performs its processes and attains its results, the more we perceive how distinctly it places in a true and just light the mutual relations and connexion of the various steps of mathematical analysis, how clearly it separates those things which are in reality distinct and independent, and unites those which are mutually dependent.

Augusta Ada Lovelace, Note B, p 706

The semantics of Receptive Process Theory, while based on the failures-divergences semantics of CSP, are simpler in that since a process cannot refuse to accept input from its environment at any time, the refusals set is simplified out of existence.

A Receptive Process is a triple (I, O, F), where I and O represent the disjoint sets of input and (non-empty) output alphabets, and may be in one of three possible states:

(1) An undesirable state, as a result of the system having engaged in a finite sequence t of inputs and outputs (i.e., a trace). The subsequent behaviour of the system is undefined, and t is a divergence of the process.
(2) A quiescent state, in which it will not output further unless it is supplied with more input.
(3) Neither undesirable nor quiescent, and hence ready to output and enter a new state.

The actual state that the process is in at any given time may be nondeterministic.

If the process is in either an undesirable or quiescent state, then the trace t is also a failure of the process, and as a consequence every divergence is a failure and every failure is a trace. That is, if $F \subseteq (I \cup O)^*$ is the set of failures of a process, and $F{\uparrow}$ and $\widehat{F}$ denote the sets of divergences and traces, respectively, of the same process, then:

$$F{\uparrow} \subseteq F \subseteq \widehat{F}.$$

In order to obtain this relationship between the sets of failures and divergences, the theory is simplified such that processes that output forever, or become quiescent in infinitely many different ways must be modelled as being in an undesirable state.

The failures-divergences model of semantics, and its associated logic system are sufficient for proof of properties of a system defined in terms of RPT.

4. RPT as a formal design method for Ada

Unlike many other design methods, formal or informal, Receptive Process theory is capable of exploiting Ada's full potential as a system development language. It provides explicit support for those features that distinguish Ada from other programming languages and so permits the design of systems involving asynchronous communication and tasking, and also supports software reuse through genericity, etc.

4.1. Asynchronous Communication

Any programming language that is to be effective for use in the development of real-time applications must support some degree of asynchronous communication. This is required in order to facilitate the reactive model of computation of which real-time systems are representative [1].

As was pointed out earlier, Ada 83 does not provide actual support for asynchronous communication, but it is anticipated that a reliable asynchronous communication primitive will be a feature of Ada 9X.

Most existing design methods do not support asynchronous communication. Two exceptions are the Theory of Asynchronous Processes [14] and JSD [12] neither of which support a truly reactive model of computation. In fact, although JSD assumes an asynchronous communication primitive, it uses this as the basis for synchronous communication which is used throughout the method.

4.2. Tasking

> *It must be evident how multifarious and how mutually complicated are the considerations which the workings of such involve. There are frequently several distinct sets of effects going on simultaneously; all in a manner independent of each other, and yet to a greater or less degree exercising a mutual influence. To adjust each to every other, and indeed even to perceive and trace them out with perfect correctness and success, entails difficulties whose nature partakes to a certain extent of those involved in every question where conditions are very numerous and inter-complicated; such as for instance the estimation of the mutual relations amongst statistical phenomena, and of those involved in many other classes of facts.*

> Augusta Ada Lovelace, Note D, p 710

Tasking is one of the features that most distinguishes Ada from other languages, and makes it so appropriate for use with real-time systems. The ability to separate and handle various tasks at once greatly simplifies the implementation of such systems.

Each distinct RPT process corresponds to an Ada task. A process is said to be 'distinct' if it is not referenced in the definition of any other process in the system. Thus the process $P = (c?m \rightarrow Q_m)$ translates into Ada as:

```
task P is
    entry C( M : in MESSAGE-TYPE );
end P;

task body P is
...
    procedure Q( M : in MESSAGE-TYPE ) is
    ...
-- Q translated
    ...
    end Q
begin
    loop
        accept C( M : in MESSAGE-TYPE ) do
            Q(M)
        end C;
    end loop;
end P;
```

Process Q would be translated in a similar manner, except that as Q is not distinct, it is translated as a procedure rather than a task. Alternatively, process Q may be expanded in-line.

Since we assume high levels of concurrency (and an infinite number of processors) when describing systems in terms of RPT, this would result in an unmanagable number of Ada tasks, which would be impractical and too expensive to implement in most environments.

This is not a problem, however, as the algebraic laws of Receptive Process Theory provide a means of reducing the number of processes in a system. If we so desire, we can reduce everything to a single process to be run in a uni-processor environment. This would obviously be an extreme move and would defeat the purpose of using Ada as the implementation language. However, it is reasonable to use the algebraic laws to produce an *equivalent* description based on a smaller number of processes (tasks).

The algebraic laws of RPT are *correctness preserving*, so (provided that the laws are applied correctly) we can be *guaranteed* that the description with a smaller number of processes is equivalent in behaviour to the highly concurrent version. In fact, taking the extreme position, and reducing everything to a single process (task) does have a benefit — it demonstrates that the distributed implementation we have described could actually be implemented as a single process and therefore increases our confidence in the implementation.

With widespread concerns over the appropriateness of Ada tasking (as it is currently defined) for use in real-time applications, this is a great benefit. In fact, reverse engineering Ada into equivalent RPT definitions could facilitate formal analysis of existing systems, and their formal manipulation (re-engineering) into equivalent systems based on a smaller number of tasks, which are known to be implementable in the context of its environmental constraints.

4.3. Exception Handling

The method fully supports multiple entry-points and the raising of exceptions.

In defining a system in Receptive Process Theory, we consider at each event the other possible events that could occur. If another event can occur, this may have a significant effect on the future behaviour of the system, and the event must be handled appropriately. Thus, each of the alternative *choices* in a process definition corresponds to various entry-points into the Ada source code.

Thus, the process P defined as:

$$P_v = (in?x \rightarrow Q_x$$
$$| c_1?x_1 \rightarrow Q1_{x_1}$$
$$| c_2?x_2 \rightarrow Q2_{x_2}$$
$$\vdots$$
$$| c_{n-1}?x_{n-1} \rightarrow QN-1_{x_{n-1}}$$
$$| c_n?x_n \rightarrow QN_{x_n}$$
$$| \quad \cdots \quad)$$

translates into Ada code as:

```
task P is
   entry IN( V : in MESSAGE-TYPE );
   entry C1( X1 : in MESSAGE-TYPE);
   entry C2( X2 : in MESSAGE-TYPE);
            . . .
   entry CN-1( XN-1 : in MESSAGE-TYPE);
   entry CN( XN : in MESSAGE-TYPE);
end P;

task body P is
. . .
   procedure Q( X : in MESSAGE-TYPE ) is
   . . .
   -- Q translated
   . . .
   end Q
begin
   loop
      select
         when i(C1) =>
            accept C1( X1 : in MESSAGE-TYPE ) do Q1(X1);
            end C1;
         or when i(C2) =>
               accept C2( X2 : in MESSAGE-TYPE) do Q2(X2);
            end C2;
```

. . . . .

```
            or when i(CN-1) =>
                  accept CN-1( XN-1 : in MESSAGE-TYPE ) do QN-1(XN-1);
                  end CN-1;
            or when i(CN) =>
                  accept CN( XN : in MESSAGE-TYPE ) do QN(XN);
                  end CN;
            or
```

. . . . .

```
         end select;
      end loop;
end P;
```

where i is the interpretation function that translates RPT events into Ada statements.

Where a *choice* corresponds to subsequent undefined behaviour (i.e., where a choice is in the format $a?b \to \bot$), it follows that either we did not expect that event to occur at that time, or that we did not expect it to occur at all. Clearly this is an exceptional event, which is to be handled by the raising of an exception. The exception handler itself can, of course, also be defined in terms of RPT if so desired.

Suppose, for example, that we are translating the non-distinct process Q into an Ada procedure, and that Q has been defined such that at a particular time the environment is obliged not to supply input on channel e. Then, Q has a definition of the format:

$$Q = (\qquad \cdots$$
$$| e?x \to \bot)$$

Input on channel e clearly requires the raising of an exception:

```
procedure Q is
    E : exception;
```

. . . . .

```
begin
```

. . . . .

```
exception
. . .

    when i(E) =>  -- handler for E (defined elsewhere)
. . .

end Q;
```

4.4.   Software Reuse

> *... A method was devised of what was technically designated* backing the
> cards in certain groups according to certain laws. *The object of this extension is
> to secure the possiblity of bringing any particular card or set of cards into use* any
> number of times successively *in the solution of one problem ...*

Augusta Ada Lovelace, Note C, p 706

The use of object-oriented techniques can greatly facilitate software reuse. Receptive
Process Theory supports such an object-oriented paradigm. Each process corresponds to
an object, responding to messages it receives on its input channels. Each process can
include the definition of other processes, and there is no limit on the number of processes
that can share any given definition.

RPT processes can then be specialized with the labelling operator. For example, [9]
describes how a button 'object' can be defined in (extended) RPT and how different
button types can be identified by appropriate labelling. Labelling is also used to identify
different instantiations. With multiple labelling, the labelling operator plays both roles.
The outermost labels distinguish the various instantiations, while the innermost labels
serve to specialize the definition.

Finally, the change of symbol operator facilitates Ada generic parameters. The operator
enables us to define processes and then use renamed versions in various specifications.
This corresponds to the derivation of a generic template in Ada, which can later be
instantiated as required. Clearly, a library of the more useful process definitions can be
built up.

5.   Future Work

Future work includes the development of a refinement calculus for the RPT to Ada
translation.

It would also be advantageous to strengthen the method by integrating RPT with a
model-based formal method such as Z [15] in order to provide greater support for non-
communication events, and hence formalize the interpretation of events as Ada statements,
i.e., function i in the above examples. This integration of Z and RPT, together with the
integration of a graphical notation, is the basis of the SB design method [16], for which
tool support is planned.

Acknowledgements

I am grateful to Dr. Mark Josephs (Oxford University PRG) for much advice and guidance,
to Professor Jack Beidler (University of Scranton) for discussions on Ada, and to Jim
Grundy (University of Cambridge) for help with typesetting.

References

1. M.G. Hinchey, The Design of Real-Time Applications, In: Proceedings of RTAW'93, 1st IEEE Workshop
    on Real-Time Applications, New York City, 11–12 May 1993, to appear, IEEE Computer Society Press,
    Los Alamitos, 1993.

2. R. Kurki-Suonio, Stepwise Design of Real-Time Systems, In: Proceedings of ACM SIGSOFT'91 Conference on Software for Critical Systems, New Orleans, 4–6 December 1991, ACM Press, New York, 1991, pp 120–131.
3. J.A. Hall, Seven Myths of Formal Methods, *IEEE Software* **7**(5) (1990), 11–19.
4. Department of Defense, DoD Trusted Computer System Evaluation Criteria.
5. Ministry of Defence, Interim Defence Standard 00-55: Requirements for the Procurement of Safety-Critical Software, 1991.
6. M.B. Josephs, Receptive Process Theory, *Acta Informatica* **29** (1992) 17–31.
7. C.A.R. Hoare, Communicating Sequential Processes, *Communications of the ACM* **21**(8) (1978) 666–677.
8. C.A.R. Hoare, Communicating Sequential Processes, Prentice-Hall International Series in Computer Science, London, 1985.
9. M.G. Hinchey, JSD, RPT & the Design of Real-Time Systems, Oxford University, Programming Research Group, September 1992.
10. J.W. Armitage & J.V. Chelini, Ada software on distributed targets: A survey of approaches, *Ada Letters* **4**(4) (1985), 32–37.
11. D.L. Dill, Trace Theory for Automatic Hierarchical Verification of Speed-Independent Circuits, MIT Press, Cambridge MA, 1989.
12. J.R. Cameron, An Overview of JSD, *IEEE Trans. on Software Engineering* **12**(2) (1986), 222–240.
13. T. Cahill & M.G. Hinchey, Systematic Disambiguation, work in progress.
14. M.B. Josephs, C.A.R. Hoare & J. He, A Theory of Asynchronous Processes, Technical Report PRG-TR-6-89, Oxford University, Programming Research Group, 1989.
15. S. Brien & J.E. Nicholls (eds.), Z Base Standard, v. 1.0, ZIP Project Report ZIP/PRG/92/121, November 1992.
16. M.G. Hinchey, Integrating Structured and Formal Methods in Real-Time Systems Design, submitted for publication.

Ada: Towards Maturity
Ed. L. Collingbourne
IOS Press 1993

From Formal Descriptions to Ada Code

P. Taylor
EDS-Scicon

Abstract

This paper gives a brief overview of the relationships between formal techniques and Ada, and considers the implications of these for when formal techniques are used in a software development lifecycle where the end product is a system implemented via Ada code. Certain aspects of this review have been made more specific by reference to the RAISE method.

1 Introduction

Formal techniques have been widely advocated for use in the software development lifecycle. Whilst formal notations provide definite advantages for presenting and analysing high-level descriptions of a system, for application it necessary that these descriptions be realised in an executable form, and specifically as Ada code. There thus exists a translation gap. In this paper we review the some of the interactions between formal techniques and Ada, which have implications for the implementation of formal specifications. Certain aspects are made more specific by consideration of how they have been approached with the RAISE method, [19].

This paper is based upon previous papers which were prepared as part of a wider project funded by the European Space Agency that is investigating the usage of formal techniques in the software development lifecycle. We would like to thank ESA for their support of this work, but would emphasise that the opinions presented here are those of the author and do not represent the policy of ESA.

2 Formal Notations and Ada

Formal methods can be used to provide a mathematical description of the functional behaviour of systems, including software systems. With formal notations, descriptions may be provided that are succinct yet unequivocal and which are susceptible to analysis via calculation and logical deduction. To achieve this, formal notations are based upon abstract concepts of mathematics and logic. Since formal notations are directed at system description and analysis, the concepts they employ are frequently not susceptible to direct execution: a formal specification may provide implicit descriptions of operations or use explicit constructions which would be highly inefficient or, for practical purposes, impossible to realise. A variety of approaches have been pursued, emphasising different approaches to system description. The selection of these being influenced by the classes of application or level of abstraction required in the description. These approaches include: model based notations (e.g Z, VDM) which employ set theoretic models; algebraic notations (e.g. OBJ, Extended ML) which use algebraic equations to express system constraints; process algebras (CCS, LOTOS), that emphasise the sequencing and co-ordination of events in the behaviour of systems; temporal logics (e.g TEMPORA), that can be used to express constraints upon evolution in time. In recent years a number of so called *Wide Spectrum* languages have been devised that combine ideas from a number of these approaches and also offer a variety of techniques for specification, suitable for use across a range of levels of abstraction, including program language style constructs. RSL, the specification language for the RAISE method, and to a lesser degree LOTOS, have been designed to be wide spectrum.

Obviously the aims of a formal description technique must overlap with those of a programming language, since both are concerned with system description. However the ultimate purpose of a programming language is to support the production of software systems, not their analysis. Thus the main objectives of the Ada language could be summarised as follows:

- To provide a set of programming constructs which are supportive of the best current practice and styles employed in conventional programming, and which are also susceptible to efficient execution upon conventional computing engines.

- To provide support for embedded control applications, that may involve parallel streams of activity and a requirement to respond effectively to externally generated events.

- Support for system development as well as program development by the provision of capabilities for building software systems from components and for the reuse and customisation of these components. These features make the construction of libraries a viable proposition, and these are indeed seen as central to the use of Ada.

The reference definition for Ada provided in [1] is expressed in English and is itself a candidate system for description via formal mathematically based notations. A formal definition of Ada is both an example of a very extensive formal specification and also a key element in the completely sound co-operative use of formal methods and Ada in the software lifecycle.

The benefits of a formal definition of Ada include the following:

- The formal definition would provide an unambiguous compiler independent reference definition of the language. This could serve as an oracle that could respond definitively to questions concerning the behaviour of Ada programs. This could be achieved by logical deduction, either manual or (ideally) machine supported, from the specification. Less ambitiously the activity of composing the formal definition should (and did) reveal areas of complexity, ambiguity or contradiction in the English description of Ada.

- A formal definition of Ada would provide a standard against which compilers could be judged. More specifically a formal definition would be an essential precursor to the development of any formally verified Ada compiler.

- It would be useful to work with Ada itself as a formal notation, for example:

  - Correctness proofs for Ada programs, require formal semantics.
  - Source to source transformation of Ada programs, require proofs of semantic equivalence of transformation schemas. This observation also holds for transformations from other formal languages to Ada.
  - Various kinds of flow analysis of Ada programs, may be defined in terms of reduced semantics of the programming language. These should be consistent with the full semantics.

Such activities are of course currently carried out, but upon a rigorous and not a formal basis.

To there have been a number of exercises in providing formal definitions for Ada, see [15, 3, 8]. Of the these the most extensive was the DDC/CRAI which covered the complete language. The resulting definition was complex covering eight volumes and employing a number of different notations, each suited to different aspects of the language. Whilst the specification exercises have been successful in clarifying the semantics of Ada and in revealing the precise nature of the complexity of the language, to a large extent the complete range of theoretical benefits identified for a formally defined language have yet to be demonstrated. This is probably due to two causes: firstly that all large scale languages designed to date have so many departures from any uniform design principles that any analysis is very difficult; and secondly, tool support for the semantics of all formal notations is still very much an area of research and viable tools have only become available in recent years.

3 Verification and Validation of Ada Code and Ada subsets

For safety critical applications it is desirable to be able confirm the quality of code in terms of the predictability and the appropriateness of its behaviour under all circumstances. Ideally this validation will not simply rely upon dynamic testing of the code, which by its very nature can only provide partial coverage of the spectrum of behaviours of the code for any non-trivial system. But should, in addition, employ static techniques for validation, which are based upon inspections of the code itself and so can provide comprehensive checking for those areas they address.

Program validation has sometimes been seen as being synonymous with providing a mathematical proof that the code accurately realises some specification. This is far from being the complete story but it is still a very strong test of quality for code. The classical approach to program correctness as originated by Floyd and Hoare [12] and most notably advanced by Dijkstra [11], is based upon the following:

1. The use of logical assertions, inserted into the program as formal comments, which characterise the dynamic state associated with the executing program at that point in the code. Such assertions, attached to the start and finish of the program, will constitute the specification of the program.

2. Rules, for each class of construction in the programming language, that characterise those pairs of assertions that can meaningfully describe the start and end states associated with the construction when it occurs within a program. This is said to be a dynamic logic or axiomatic semantics for the programming language.

For Ada there have been no completely successful attempts at providing a dynamic logic. A notable piece of work in this area is the Anna project [17]. The key aspect of this project was the provision of formal comments (introduced by the string --: or --| in contrast to to the usual --) for annotating the Ada programs. The Anna tool can use these comments in validation of Ada programs, by compiling them and executing them along with the actual code to check that the states reached by the program conform to the constraints specified by the comments. The Anna language added specification facilities consistent with a large proportion of the Ada language (tasking features were not dealt with), and was proposed as being the appropriate specification language for use with Ada. (The Asphodel language [13] was also proposed as specification extension to Ada). However providing the axiomatic semantics for Anna and suitable tools to support formal proof appears to have been less successful. Indeed the rich mix of features that is present in Ada presents difficulties to the construction of a complete axiomatic semantics for Ada, see for instance [7].

In validating programs other static analysis techniques, weaker in content than full formal proof but more susceptible to automation than complete proof have been applied. These include:

- Control, data and information flow analysis.

- Call graph analysis.

- Storage requirements analysis.

- Interval analysis.

- Exception analysis.

It is interesting to note that an Ada program might still be formally correct and yet be unsuitable for a critical application because of its violation of other less functional requirements, for instance its profligate use of storage, its tardy execution time or the access it allows to confidential data. Non-conformance to such requirements can sometimes be detected by these weaker static analysis techniques. However specifying even these tests requires a good understanding of the formal semantics of a language and is accordingly difficult to achieve completely for full Ada.

In view of the complexity of the semantics of full Ada, subsets have been proposed for use in critical applications. Such 'safe' subsets retain some of the support for good software engineering practice that Ada provides, whilst omitting those features of the language whose semantics are problematic or whose performance requirements are difficult to predict. One of the more well known subsets is the SPARK [1] Ada subset [5], which has been mandated for the safety critical code used on the European Fighter Aircraft. The main exclusions from Ada in SPARK are:

- tasks,

- exceptions,

- generics,

- derived types other than numeric types,

- dynamic storage objects including access types, dynamic arrays, discriminants, and recursion,

- default expressions and mixed positional/name parameter passing,

- overloading of names and restriction of renaming and use clause.

---

[1]SPARK is a trade mark of Program Validation Ltd

The SPARK Examiner tool [6] is available which provides support for data and information flow analysis and formal correctness proofs of SPARK code. A formal semantics for SPARK is being developed in Z and it has been suggested that the level of complexity of SPARK is such that the implementation of a formally verified compiler is potentially feasible with current techniques.

Finally it should be observed that having a verified compiler is only one link in the chain of entities involved in the actual execution of any code, e.g. there is an operating system, an assembler for the machine code, the actual computer itself. With the current development of technology it is difficult to see how such complete verification could achieved for actual systems or to argue that the benefits would justify the costs. To date the most extensive attempt in build a verified stack, but not for Ada, has been carried out by Computational Logic Co., see [20].

4   Formal Development to Ada

In recent years it has become increasingly accepted that the best approach to implementing a system starting from a formal presentation of its requirements is via processes of refinement, where a sequence of system specifications is produced that identify, with increasing explicitness, the details of the implementation. It is within this paradigm of development that wide spectrum formal techniques fit, since they offer notations suited to the description of all the levels of abstraction. Refinement may be seen as offering a viewpoint on system development that unifies the insights provided by both formal program verification techniques (in that each specification has to be proved consistent with it proceeding specification) and hierarchical design techniques [14] (in that each level of specification adds detail to the previous specifications). However the formal notion of refinement is very flexible since the structure of one specification doesn't have to constrain the structure of the succeeding specification only its behaviour.

A formal notion of refinement requires compositional operations for combining specifications. This means that the specifications of components may be refined independently but when a fitted together they will still provide the behaviour required for the complete system.

System development by refinement is the approach advocated by the RAISE method and we shall orient much of the following discussion to this approach. Parallel arguments could also be given for other wide spectrum formal notations, see for instance the papers in [4] for an indication of the current situation for LOTOS. In the RAISE method, refinements are recorded in development relations.

Verification and validation of a system developed by a formal refinement process is achieved by a number of activities, each of which should ideally be supported by computer based tools. Areas for verification and validation, as a minimum, should include:

- Validating that the top level system specification is internally consistent and conformant with the informal requirements of the user.

- Verifying that each level of specification is consistent with the specification from which it was derived, in that it satisfies the constraints imposed or displays an equivalent behaviour when observed at an appropriate level of abstraction.

- Verifying the correctness of the transformation of the low level specification into an executable format, such as Ada code.

Each of these validation requirements must be met in somewhat different way.

Validating that a specification meets a customer's requirements is the most difficult to achieve, since by their very nature these may be loosely conceived and open ended in their achievement. Essentially the specification can be used as the basis for a dialogue with the customer. By inspection and review, questions can raised from or asked of the specification. Such questions may be very general, relating to global properties of the specification, or they may be very specific queries, such as which outputs should occur in response to particular inputs. In this situation the fact that the specification is formal means that answers, if they can be deduced, will be unambiguous. In questioning a specification, the fact that it is a mathematical object means that sometimes answers can be calculated from the specification, i.e. the specification can be animated.

Verifying consistency between a specification and its refinement is a precisely defined activity. Firstly this requires the generation of a finite collection of formal verification conditions and then demonstrating that each of these holds. Demonstrating that a verification condition holds can vary from being a simple integrity check that each operation of the original specification has an interpretation and is provided with an appropriate data typing in the refined specification, to proving some mathematical property.

Verifying translations ought to be similar in scope to verifying refinements, but since a language boundary is being crossed it is much more problematic. Theoretically what is required is that the semantics of the implementation should be expressed within the formalism of the specification language and then the translation can be seen as a reformulation of the original specification and a proof of equivalence could be given. However, as has been noted earlier, formalising the semantics of a language as complex as Ada presents a considerable challenge. At the moment perhaps the best that can be achieved is to rely on the ability of the experts, designing the schemes for translation, to identify interpretations of the semantics that are valid in the majority of circumstances. Of course these transformations can be tested by executing the resulting code.

What is obvious from the discussions above is that substantial tool support is required for the systematic use of a formal method, not simply for the syntax and type checking but also for exploring the semantics of the formal notation. Support tools for RAISE were developed along with the formal notation and the methodology for its use, and a fairly comprehensive tool set is now available, [2] see [16].

The RAISE tool set has four major components:

- A Module editor for RSL (RAISE Specification Language) that provides built in syntax and type checking.

- Support for the use and maintenance of libraries of RSL modules.

- A Justification editor to support proof of properties of specifications and verification conditions for refinements.

- Translators from RSL to Ada and C++.

---

[2] The RAISE tools are marketed by Computer Resources International,CRI

Of these the last two have the most significance for verification and validation of specifications and refinements, although checking of the static consistency of refinements is carried out by what is essentially a specialised form of the Module editor.

The justification editor is an interactive editor for proofs about RSL specifications and development relations. Essentially the editor provides the means for applying the various proof rules that define the properties of RSL. However a theorem can be justified to various levels of rigour (hence a justification editor), from a comment that makes a simple assertion of its truth to an elaboration in complete detail of all the steps necessary to establish formal truth. Depending upon the way it is used, the rules it applies and the way it applies these rules, the justification editor provides a range of functionalities. These include

- A general proof capability for theorems relating to specifications and verification conditions of development relations.

- Generation and automatic proof (to some extent) of confidence conditions for RSL specifications. Confidence conditions are simple well-formedness properties of specifications, that require more than type checking to validate; for instance that a function call always takes an argument from its domain subtype.

- Generation of the verification conditions for a development relation. In practice the assertion that one specification is a refinement of another is simply another kind of theorem requiring proof and the editor has built in rules which expand out the implications of this.

- Animation of specifications by the simplification of expressions. Essentially the editor provides a mechanism for symbolic evaluation; this is a by-product of a general capability (simplification) required for proof. This is not the most efficient approach to animation, but is in principle applicable to the whole language.

An alternative to symbolic evaluation for animation of a specification is rapid prototyping, that is translating to an executable language. Since this is not making direct use of the specification language, prototyping is potentially less comprehensive and less sound than symbolic evaluation; however in practice it seems to have provided the easiest approach to animation. RAISE tools provide translators to C++ and Ada, these languages being appropriate for RSL which is very modular and promotes an object oriented style of specification.

The RAISE Ada translator will take a RSL file containing a specification module and produce a compilation unit containing an Ada package and potentially some auxiliary packages, a list of the dependencies and the order in which they should be compiled. The translator will preserve the genericity of the RAISE specifications, in that if the original RSL module was parameterised then the Ada package produced by translation will be generic.

The translation function was intended to be as comprehensive as possible so as to provide the widest scope for early prototyping, whilst at the same time not unduly restricting the direction that a development should take. Thus translation is available for: explicit definitions of functions and sets; the imperative programming style constructs of RSL (i.e. variables, assignments, conditionals and loops); and the modularisation constructs. The major omissions from the translator are with respect to: implicit styles of specification using postconditions and logical quantifiers like "Exists" and "Forall; and in relation to the concurrency modelling features of RSL, for which there are no obvious and at the same time acceptably efficient translation to Ada. Extension to concurrent constructs is however planned. Further discussion of the details of translator may be found in [16, 9]

As noted previously the translator was provided originally for early prototyping and animation of specifications. As a result the translations aim at generality and give rise to unexpected and inefficient implementations in certain situations. For example a data item represented in a specification as a mapping ranging over a small set of integers would probably be most usefully implemented via an array, however the translator's general construction employs a linked list. Nevertheless in this prototyping role and for non-challenging environments, the code produced by the translators has proved to be effective, see [2]. (Wider experience with using RAISE and the Ada translator is being accumulated in the LACOS project [10].) Moreover the translator provides the overall package structure for an implementation, so that if a more optimised implementation is required, then certain modules may be replaced by hand coded packages. This approach has proved to be effective in practice and it is planned to enhance the translator so that it can support this style of usage more directly [18]. Thus the translator can supply the basis for an implementation, but in view of such efficiency considerations and the fact that the translations are intuitively plausible but not formally proven, they should not be used in critical applications without additional verification of the code by conventional techniques. Of course since the code has been automatically generated it will be uniform in style and liable to present fewer problems in analysis than hand coded Ada.

5 Conclusions

Formal methods can vastly enhance the rigour with which the requirements capture and design phases of a software development may be executed, by providing means of system description that are much more precise and analysable than those of pragmatically derived techniques currently in widespread use. However the features which provide this advantage, namely their mathematical foundations, imply that much firmer criteria must be identified for their valid use. This in turn implies that more sophisticated tool support is also desirable. Thus, although formal methods ought to be widely applied in software engineering, their integration into contemporary practice has involved a long and continuing learning curve. Formal techniques, such as LOTOS and RAISE, having sound theoretical foundations but which can also be applied effectively to the description of real systems and have suitable tool support, have only recently become available.

Today, moderate scale developments may be tackled formally. Moreover for larger systems it can be worthwhile to analyse and/or formally develop certain properties or subsystems of larger systems. However with critical systems a "belt and braces" approach should be followed, so that whilst the formal techniques may be used to provide increased understanding and confidence about a system and its implementation, conventional validation techniques must also be applied for a basic degree of assurance. Thus automatically generated code should be reviewed and tested as carefully as that generated manually. (However the errors arising within an automatic tool should be consistent and once removed from the tool should not reoccur). Since the code for real applications must satisfy numerous non-functional requirements (e.g. performance concerns, user interface considerations), it must be anticipated that such dual validation will, in some form, continue to be required into the foreseeable future.

Today it is clear that there are many complementary aspects to software engineering, and that software development environments should allow the mutually supportive use of a range of tools and techniques. Consequently whilst formal techniques may lie at the technical base of a software development, tools to support planning, management and product assurance must also be available for use with such techniques. The ESA project, mentioned earlier, is investigating these issues in the context of LOTOS and RAISE and a particular software development environment, the ESSDE (European Space Software Development Environment).

Verification and validation is one of the key issues in software development, and in the longer term should be central to the design of future programming and specification languages. Thus the design of a programming language should also involve the construction of the various associated formal semantics. Whilst a wide spectrum specification language should be designed with sublanguages explicitly orientated towards implementation, perhaps some would resemble safe Ada subsets.

6 Acknowledgements

The author would like to thank ESA for their support of this work via their funding of the Advanced Methods and Tools in ESSDE Project. EDS-Scicon's subcontractors in this project are BSO, CRI, CRISA, ITA and UPM. The author in particular wishes to thank Jan Pedersen of CRI for discussions with respect to the philosophy of RAISE and its tools.

References

[1]   ANSI/MIL-STD-1815A-1983: Reference Manual For The Ada Programming Language, 1983

[2]   Alapide A, Cinnella M, and La Vopa P.: Automatic Generation of Ada Code with the RAISE formal method. Proceedings Ada in Aerospace 1992.

[3]   Bjørner D. and Oest O.: Towards a Formal Description of Ada, LNCS Vol 98, Springer 1980.

[4]   Bolognesi T., Brinksma E., and Vissers C. *eds*: Proceedings of 3rd LotosSphere Workshop, Pisa 1992

[5]   Carré B. A, Jennings T. J, Maclennan F. J., Farrow, P. F, and Garnsworthy J. R: SPARK – The SPADE Ada Kernel, Program Validation Limited Report, Third Edition, 1990.

[6]   Carré B., Garnsworthy J.: SPARK - An Annotated Ada Subset for Safety Critical Programming, ACM Tri-Ada Conference, Baltimore, December 1990.

[7]   Cohen N.: Ada Axiomatic Semantics: Problems and Solutions, *in* Ada: managing the transition, CUP 1986.

[8]   DDC/CRAI: The Draft Formal Definition of Ada, DDC/CRAI87

[9]   Dandanall B.: Fast and Rigorous Prototyping in Ada, Proceedings Ada in Aerospace 1991.

[10]   Dandanall B. and George C.: The LaCoS Project, LaCoS and CRI 1991.

[11]   Dijkstra E.: A Discipline of Programming, Prentice Hall 1976.

[12]   Hoare C.A.R.: An Axiomatic basis for computer programming, *in* Comms ACM 12, 1969.

[13]   Hill, A: The Formal Specification and Verification of Reusable Software Components Using Ada With Asphodel, Technical Report, 1987.

[14]   HOOD User Group: HOOD Reference Manual, release 3.1, HUG and Prentice Hall 1992.

[15]   INRIA: Formal Definition of the Ada Programming Language, CII Honeywell Bull 1982.

[16]   LaCoS Consortium: RAISE Tools Reference Manual, LaCoS and CRI 1992.

[17]   Luckham D. C, von Henke, F. W, Krieg-Brueckner B, and Owe, O: ANNA, A Language for Annotating Ada Programs, Lecture Notes in Computer Science No. 260, Springer-Verlag, 1987.

[18]   Pedersen J.: Email communication, 1993.

[19]   The RAISE Language Group: The RAISE Specification Language, Prentice Hall 1992.

[20]   Young W.: Verified Program Support Environments, *in* Proceedings ACM SIG-SOFT Workshop on Formal Methods in Software Development, ACM 1990

Ada: Towards Maturity
Ed. L. Collingbourne
IOS Press 1993

Worst-case timing analysis of exception handling in Ada

Roderick Chapman, Alan Burns, Andy Wellings

British Aerospace Dependable Computing Systems Centre,
Department of Computer Science, University of York,
York, U.K.

Abstract. This paper describes a method for analysing the timing properties of exception handling in Ada. The paper first describes how exceptions are implemented and considers the use of exceptions in the SPARK, Safe/Ada and ANNA subsets. A static analysis technique for reasoning about exception propagation is then presented. We argue that this technique, along with a suitable subset and detailed knowledge of exception implementation can be used to develop an accurate worst-case timing analysis system. The method is illustrated with an example. Finally, our conclusions and plans for further work are presented.

1. Introduction

Hard real-time systems are characterised by their need to meet stringent timing requirements. The application of static analysis techniques to determine the worst-case execution time of program fragments has therefore become an important topic. Knowledge of worst-case execution times is essential if schedulability analysis is to be used to guarantee an application's timing properties. Research in this field has concentrated on three topics: computer architecture, language design, and static analysis methods. The latter two topics complement each other: a language-subset for hard real-time programming must be large enough to express useful programs, but small enough to allow efficient and accurate static analysis.

In the development of a subset of Ada that is amenable to static timing analysis, certain language features have to be excluded. Access types, recursive subprograms, and unbounded loops are typical of this class since they generally have unbounded or unpredictable execution time. Current timing analysis tools[1-3] have imposed rather Draconian restrictions, only allowing the simplest language constructs. Exceptions are undoubtedly a useful feature of Ada, but they are currently beyond the capabilities of contemporary timing analysis tools. This paper therefore focuses on the development of an analysable subset and static analysis method for exceptions in Ada.

In section 2 the implementation of the current exception handling facilities in Ada83 is discussed. It is assumed that the reader is at least familiar with the general style of exception handling in Ada. By considering the implementation of exceptions, difficulties in their analysis are highlighted. The approaches to exception handling taken in three Ada subsets are also detailed here.

Section 3 considers how static analysis techniques can be applied to allow reasoning about exception handling. One such technique "Exception flow analysis" is described in detail. Section 4 proposes a subset of Ada exceptions suitable for use in hard real-time systems and describes our approach for their analysis. Finally, section 5 presents our conclusions and plans for further work.

2. Exception handling in Ada83

Before the timing analysis of exceptions is considered, we must understand how exceptions are implemented in Ada83. The four central topics are: how exceptions are detected, raised, handled and propagated. Within each of these areas, an Ada implementation has a certain amount of freedom - the trade-offs of time, space, complexity, etc. apply here as usual. The sections below look at each of the standard implementation techniques, concentrating on their impact upon timing analysis. A more detailed description is given by Baker and Riccardi[4].

2.1. Detecting exceptions

The job of detecting whether an exception must be raised can be subdivided into the following cases:
- Predefined exceptions, implicitly detected.
- Predefined exceptions, detected by runtime checks.
- User defined exceptions.

The first of these classes is the set of predefined exceptions that are detected automatically at runtime by the target computer system. These include the classic cases of divide-by-zero and memory-faults. These are detected by the hardware and are treated as processor exceptions or "traps." The Ada runtime system must then detect these traps and translate them into the appropriate Ada exception.

The second case is simpler. These are the predefined exceptions raised by runtime checks (such as ACCESS_CHECK or INDEX_CHECK) as defined in the Ada LRM. The rules regarding the generation of these runtime checks are complex. Indeed, an implementation is allowed a great deal of freedom in eliminating and optimising checks. Fortunately, the policy employed by the compiler for check generation is largely separate from the mechanisms used to raise and handle the actual exceptions.

User defined exceptions are raised explicitly with a raise statement and so are detected by purposely designed code.

2.2. Raising exceptions

The job of raising an exception in a task usually falls to the Ada runtime system. Most implementations use a mechanism by which an exception is "posted" to a task by the runtime system in response to a hardware trap, a check failure, or a raise statement. The important point is that each exception has its own identifier. Some implementations use integers for exception identifiers, some use pointers to the exception's name - the choice here is wide and really does not matter as long as the identifiers are distinct. When the task is next scheduled to run, the outstanding exception is detected and exception handling is initiated. We therefore come to exception handling itself.

2.3. Exception handling

This section is concerned with how the exception handlers are compiled and executed at runtime. An implementation has a little freedom here; the two most popular choices are the *compiled handlers* approach and the *table based* approach. These are illustrated below with an example.

Consider the following simple exception handler:

```
exception
   when A I B =>
          STM1;
   when C =>
          STM2;
   when others =>
          STM3;
end;
```

The *compiled* approach translates this handler into a simple *if* or *case* statement, thus:

```
declare
   E : EXCEPTION_IDENTIFIER :=
          CURRENT_EXCEPTION;
begin
   if (E = A) or (E = B) then
          STM1;
   elsif (E = C) then
          STM2;
   else
          STM3;
   end if;
end;
```

The *table* approach, on the other hand, would translate the handler's structure into a table of exception identifiers and the addresses of the code for each arm of the handler. This table is then interpreted by a runtime system routine that searches the table and performs an indirect jump to the correct handler. The table and compiled code would look something like this:

Exception ID	Handler address
A	LAB1
B	LAB1
C	LAB2
others	LAB3

```
<<LAB1>>      STM1;
              goto ENDLAB;
<<LAB2>>      STM2;
              goto ENDLAB;
<<LAB3>>      STM3;
<<ENDLAB>>
```

For timing analysis, either approach can be analysed - both approaches mirror the possible implementations of a simple case statement. Timing analysis for these situations is well-understood[5].

2.4. Exception propagation

The major complexity in Ada83 exceptions occurs when no handler can be found in the current frame - the exception must then be propagated to the enclosing frames, searching for a handler in each. The main problem is that when subprogram calls are traversed, the propagation is based upon the *dynamic* call sequence of frames, not on their lexical nesting. This feature has two important consequences:

- The handler to which an exception will propagate cannot be determined statically.
- The handler must be searched for at runtime by "unwinding" the dynamic call chain.

The most popular mechanism for doing this stores information in the tasks' activation records about the "closest" enclosing frame with an exception handler. These records are linked in the same style as the dynamic-link used to maintain the stack. When an exception is raised, the closest handler is executed - if no matching handler can be found, the link is followed to the next frame with a handler and so on. These actions are accompanied by the normal actions of cleaning up the stack, local storage, and the heap as each frame is exited. This scheme has the advantages of simple implementation and fast exception handling. Its main drawback is the overhead associated with maintaining the dynamic chain of handlers on the stack. This overhead is always incurred (whether exceptions are ever raised or not) and so is not favoured by some users and implementors.

The other popular scheme is to build a global table containing ordered pairs of values. The first value gives the program-counter's value for the start of the code for each frame. The second value gives the address of the nearest handler that must be executed if an exception is raised when the PC is between the given value and the next PC value in the table. Exception handling is achieved by searching the table with the current PC value as a key and executing the given handler. Exceptions are propagated by unwinding the stack (thus yielding the calling frame's PC value) and repeating the operation. This scheme has the advantage of imposing no overhead at runtime on code which does not raise exceptions, but is complicated by the need to build the exception tables statically (this requires a special Ada linker that can build tables for an entire program taking into account the exact structure of compilation units and their relocation etc.) There are a few variations on this theme (e.g. having the table unsorted, or having both high and low PC values for each frame in the table), but they are all essentially equivalent.

In terms of timing analysis, the need to propagate exceptions is a major problem. To simply ban propagation from an Ada subset would severely limit the usefulness of exceptions as a whole. Some subset is required that allows useful programs to be written, but still allows static analysis. The next sections, then, consider what approach existing Ada subsets have taken to exceptions.

2.5. Exception handling in Ada subsets

As stated above, this section considers how existing Ada subsets handle exceptions (if at all).

2.5.1. Exceptions without tasking

If the tasking constructs are removed from the language, then the implementation of exceptions is greatly simplified. Without tasking, the runtime-system routines needed to handle and propagate exceptions are much simpler (mainly owing to the absence of the abort statement and the complex exception handling when tasks are engaged in a rendezvous).

2.5.2. SPARK

The SPARK Ada subset[6] totally excludes exceptions. SPARK's designers argue that user-defined exceptions should not be needed and that the predefined exceptions should never be raised in a well-constructed program. They also cite the lack of a formal definition of exceptions as a reason for their exclusion. We should remember that the major goals of SPARK (formal definition and proof) force different decisions from those that might be taken if a subset was developed with only timing analysis in mind.

2.5.3. Safe/Ada

The goals of the Safe Ada subset [7] are slightly different from those of SPARK. Safe Ada does not stress formal definition and proof to the same extent as SPARK: the Safe Ada subset is therefore significantly larger than SPARK. In the area of exception handling, Safe Ada imposes the following restrictions:
1) An exception shall not be propagated out of its scope.
2) An exception handler shall not have an others choice.
3) Actions shall not raise a predefined exception.
4) Subprograms shall not be called recursively.
5) Tasks and tasking statements shall not be used.

This subset bans predefined exceptions (point 3) but does allow a well-controlled subset of user-defined exceptions to be used. With respect to timing, the Safe Ada language definition notes:

"After an exception E (e.g. by `raise E;`) the dynamic subprogram call chain must be searched backward in order to find an exception handler for E. The maximum number of steps within this search is the maximum number of nested subprogram calls that can occur in the program at run time. The nesting depth is limited by excluding recursive calls from Safe Ada."

This approach does indeed place an upper bound on the exception handling time, but says nothing about how such a bound could be determined.

2.5.4. ANNA

The ANNA language[8] is an extended version of Ada intended to support the formal specification of the intended behaviour of a program. These specifications are written as annotations in a program's source text. They support the formal specification of a program's behaviour through the traditional style of predicate logic preconditions, postconditions and assertions. The ANNA language supports almost the entire Ada language - the principle exclusion is tasking. Of particular interest to us in this context are the annotations used to describe exception propagation.

ANNA includes two types of annotation to specify the propagation of exceptions. The first type is known as a *strong propagation annotation*. These are applied to the specification of a subprogram and have the form:

```
--| Boolean_expression => raise exception_name
```

In short, a strong annotation is used to specify which conditions on input parameters will lead to an exception being raised As an example, consider the following specification of a PUSH subprogram in a traditional STACK package:

procedure PUSH (E : **in** ITEM; STACK : **in out** STACK_TYPE);
--| **where in** STACK.LENGTH = SIZE => **raise** OVERFLOW,

This specifies that if the *in* parameter STACK.LENGTH = SIZE (where SIZE is some visible constant) then the subprogram *must* propagate the OVERFLOW exception to the caller. While the strong annotation is used to specify which exceptions must be raised according to the *input* parameters of a call, a *weak* annotation is used to specify the state of the *output* parameters after an exception is propagated. Continuing the example above, we could extend the strong annotation with the following weak annotation:

--| **raise** OVERFLOW => STACK = **in** STACK;

This annotation specifies that if OVERFLOW is propagated, then the state given in the assertion holds in the caller (e.g. that the STACK parameter is unchanged). Both weak and strong annotations may also be applied to any single statement and to the code executing in the elaboration of a declarative part. Any number of such annotations can be used, although the Boolean expressions in a set of strong annotations should, of course, be mutually exclusive. If they were not, then they would specify that more than one exception could be raised simultaneously - this is not possible in Ada. Similarly, the exceptions mentioned in a series of weak annotations must be distinct.

The ANNA annotations offer a powerful and flexible notation for describing exception occurrence and propagation. In particular, both annotations can be used to express that predefined exceptions can be raised by a piece of code (when it is not obvious from the source code). Such an annotation would be needed in timing analysis, since assuming that predefined exceptions could be raised anywhere would be ridiculously pessimistic. There is also the possibility that such annotations could be verified automatically; the exception flow analysis described below could be used to confirm user-supplied annotations. Strong annotations are potentially very useful for timing analysis since they effectively provide a condition under which control-flow through a block is limited to raise a particular exception. Weak annotations are also useful, since they specify a state to which a program must return after handling a possibly unexpected exception.

3. Exception flow analysis

This section considers the sole technique[9] that has been proposed for the static analysis of Ada exceptions. Baker and Sutton realise that the flow of exceptions is, in some ways, analogous to the flow of data in a program. Their technique is therefore based upon the traditional dataflow analysis techniques performed by many optimising compilers.

Their tool allows common errors to be found, such as exceptions that can be propagated out of the scope of the main program. More complex queries can also be answered, such as "Which exceptions do not have a handler in their immediately enclosing scope?" These types of queries are particularly useful for timing analysis, since they allow the limits of exception propagation to be checked.

3.1. The exception flow technique

Baker and Sutton's technique has the following ingredients:
1) The "unit" of analysis is an *exception context*. A context is one of: a package declaration, package body, task declaration, task body, subprogram body, block statement, or an accept statement. The context is therefore the Ada constructs with which exceptions can be associated and handled. It is roughly analogous to the idea of a basic-block used in dataflow analysis.
2) Instead of the program control-flow graph, exception flow analysis deals with the *context graph*. This is formed from the union of three relations between the contexts:
   i)   The *contains* relation. A context C_1 contains a context C_2 if C_2 is lexically enclosed in C_1 and is at the outermost lexical level in C_1. This relation reflects the immediate lexical nesting of contexts in the program's source code.
   ii)   The *calls* relation. C_1 calls C_2 if C_1 contains a subprogram call or entry call of the subprogram or accept statement represented by C_2 at the outermost lexical level within its sequence of statements.
         Both these relations are constrained by the allowable syntactic nesting of contexts (for example, accept statements can only contain other accepts or block statements).
   iii) The closure of the "withs" relation between compilation units. This is needed to deal with exceptions that occur during library-unit elaboration.
The context graph is therefore represented as a triple (S, N, E) where N is the set of contexts, E is the set of directed edges formed by the union of the three relations described above, and S is the start or "entry" node in N. S effectively models the environment-task of the main Ada program.

The traditional "live variable" problem in dataflow analysis has an equivalent "live exception" problem. Baker draws an analogy between the definition and use of variables and the handling and raising of exceptions. The traditional live variable problem, thus:

"A variable v is *live* at the bottom of a node i if and only if there is a definition-free path from i to a use of v in some node j below i in the flow graph."

can be restated for exceptions:

"An exception v is live at the bottom of a node i if and only if there is a handler-free path from i to a raise of v in some node j below i in the context graph."

Remember that exceptions only "flow" one way - "up" the context graph, reflecting the dynamic and lexical nesting of the contexts. Baker's solution to this problem is expressed using the following sets:

LEBOT(i)	Exceptions which are live at the bottom of context i. This can be informally defined as the set of exceptions that can be propagated into context i from contexts "below" i in the context graph.
HANDLED(i)	The set of exceptions that have a handler in context i.
RAISED(i)	The set of exceptions that are raised in context i.

The sets HANDLED(i) and RAISED(i) can be computed statically from a program's source code. The solution to the "live exceptions" problem for each node is therefore given by the smallest set LEBOT(i) that satisfies the following equation:

$$LEBOT(i) = \bigcup_{j \in succ(i)} \left[(LEBOT(j) \cup RAISED(j)) - HANDLED(j) \right] \qquad (1)$$

where succ(i) is the set of successor nodes of i in the context graph.

Baker and Sutton suggest an iterative algorithm for the solution of this equation. RAISED and HANDLED are first constructed from the raise statements and exception handlers in the source code. A "when others" handler needs a special value representing "all exceptions" in the HANDLED set, since a "when others" effectively kills all exceptions that propagate into such a handler. The context-graph is then traversed bottom-up, building LEBOT repeatedly until no further change is recorded. Once LEBOT is computed, the following types of query can be answered:

1) Which exceptions can be propagated out of the main program? (i.e. which exceptions are live at the bottom of the start context S?)

2) Which handlers are unnecessary? (i.e. are there any handlers in a context in which the handled exception can never be raised or propagated?)

3) Which exceptions can possibly appear at the top of the handler part of each context? This query is answered by forming the union of the LEBOT and RAISED sets for the given context.

4) In recursion-free programs, how many times can an exception be propagated before it is handled? This type of question is handled by tracing the appearance of an exception in the LEBOT sets "up" the context graph from the point where it is raised, to the point where it is finally handled.

3.2. Problems with exception flow analysis

This technique, although useful, has several problems. These are summarised below.

- The handling of tasks is difficult. The propagation of exceptions during rendezvous has to be carefully handled. Task types and task-access types mean that a separate context has to be created for each possible instance of a task type.

- The technique assumes that predefined exceptions can be raised almost anywhere. A more accurate analysis is needed - considering the types of statements in a context, for example, would allow some predefined exceptions to be eliminated from consideration.

- The technique assumes that all control paths are executable. This makes the results somewhat pessimistic. The results could be improved by using some other static analysis system to eliminate unexecutable paths.

- The automated (e.g. by an optimiser) or manual (e.g. pragma SUPPRESS) elimination of checks is not considered.

- Generic units cannot be analysed "as is" - they have to be handled on a per-instantiation basis.

- The "when others" and anonymous-raise constructs are difficult to handle. The when-others effectively kills all live exceptions entering a context. A raise in a handler effectively "resurrects" them.

Unfortunately, this work was never followed up[10] so none of the above problems were resolved. We feel, though, that these ideas offer a useful basis for developing a static analysis technique for reasoning about the propagation of exceptions.

4. Timing analysis of exceptions

This section considers how timing analysis of exceptions can be performed. First, a model of the control flow of exceptions is developed. From this, a scheme to analyse their timing is derived. We start by considering the language subset.

- Our base is the SPARK Ada subset[6]. SPARK's goals (formal definition, logical soundness, amenability to formal proof, bounded space and time etc.) make it ideal as a base for a worst-case execution time analysis system.
- We plan to re-introduce exceptions to SPARK with the following restrictions:
  1) Recursion remains forbidden.
  2) The "when others" and anonymous raise constructs are banned since they are troublesome for both exception flow and timing analysis. Explicit raise statements inside handlers are also forbidden.
  3) Initialising expressions in declarative sections are banned as in SPARK Ada. This eliminates the possibility of exceptions being raised during elaboration.
  4) We inherit the weak propagation annotation from ANNA. This allows the programmer to indicate where predefined exceptions may be raised.

We now have the ingredients necessary to develop a timing analysis method for exceptions. Consider a program's control flow for a simple frame of code. A *frame* is defined to be any Ada construct which can have an exception *handler* (e.g. a block statement, subprogram body, and so on). Note that this is a subset of the definition of a context used in section 3.1. In the simplest case, we can consider a frame in which no exceptions can ever be raised or a frame in which all exceptions are handled locally. The control-flow graph for such a frame is shown in figure one.

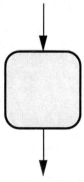

Figure 1

The worst case execution time (or WCET) for such a frame is given by summing the worst case execution times of its statements and so on. Note that this frame has a single entry point and a single exit. This property allows the WCET to be determined *once* for the frame in isolation. This WCET value is then used whenever the frame is called by other frames, subprograms and so on. If we consider the frame in more detail, we discover that Ada imposes a certain internal structure to the code of a frame. There is an optional *prologue*, the *code* itself, the *handler* part, and the *epilogue.* The prologue is concerned with allocating local storage for the frame (such as the activation record) and any other required actions such as the elaboration of the declarative section of the frame. The epilogue is concerned with deallocating local storage and reclaiming heap space used in the frame (either implicitly or via access types) and any other actions that may be needed as the frame is left. For simplicity, we assume that the handler part and the code share the same epilogue. The diagram of the frame is shown in figure two:

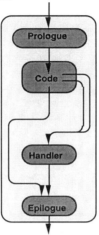

Figure 2

When all exceptions are handled locally (as shown in the diagram by control arcs from the middle of the code to the handler), then the WCET can still be determined statically. A naive approach would be to use the following equation:

$$
\begin{aligned}
WCET(frame) = {} & WCET(prologue) + \\
& WCET(code) + WCPT + \\
& WCFINDT + WCET(handler) + \\
& WCET(epilogue)
\end{aligned} \tag{2}
$$

where

WCPT is the worst case time to *post* an exception.

WCFINDT is the worst case time to find the handler. In the "compiled handlers" implementation, WCFINDT actually corresponds to the time taken to execute the if/elsif parts of the handler. In the static-tables implementation, WCFINDT is the time needed to search the global exception table.

This analysis is not realistic. In particular, this equation ignores two important points:

1) The raising of an exception is effectively a non-returning "goto" to the exception handler. The code "after" a raise is never executed.

2) In response to each exception that can be raised in a frame, only *one* unique handler is executed.

Consider a simple example: a single exception is raised somewhere in the above *code* section. We can therefore ignore code following the raise in that particular case. This requires some new notation to express the exclusion of code following a raise statement:

$$
WCET(statement - sequence) \atop {\scriptstyle raise\,E}
$$

This notation refers to the worst-case execution time for the statement-sequence up to and including the *raise* of exception E. A new notation for the WCET of handlers is also needed:

$$WCET_{E\_ID=E}(handler - part)$$

This denotes the worst case execution time for the handler given that the exception identity E is known. This limits the control-flow to a single handler. To construct the WCET for the whole frame, then, we also need to know the set of exceptions, RAISED, that can be raised in the *code* part of the frame. When an exception can be raised more than once in a frame, it must be considered once for each possible raise. This means that each raise of each exception must be given a unique value in the RAISED set. The set difference operator "-" has to be modified so that a single handler for an exception kills *all* occurrences of that exception. For example, consider a frame **i** which can raise CONSTRAINT-ERROR in four different places. For timing analysis, we need to consider each of these individually, so we have:

$$RAISED(i) = \{CONSTRAINT\_ERROR_1,$$
$$CONSTRAINT\_ERROR_2,$$
$$CONSTRAINT\_ERROR_3,$$
$$CONSTRAINT\_ERROR_4\}$$

If this frame has a single handler for *any* occurrence of CONSTRAINT_ERROR, then we require the "-" operator to "kill" all four of the above exceptions, i.e:

$$RAISED(i) - \{CONSTRAINT\_ERROR\} = \varnothing$$

The WCET for the frame is therefore given by considering the maximum of the non-exception raising path and each of the paths executed for each possible exception. WCET(frame) is therefore given by:

$$WCET(frame) = WCET(prologue) + WCET(epilogue) +$$

$$\max \left[\begin{array}{l} WCET(code) \\ \max_{\forall E:E \subseteq RAISED} \left(\begin{array}{l} WCET(code) + WCPT + \\ {\scriptstyle raise\ E} \\ WCFINDT + WCET_{E\_ID=E}(handler) \end{array} \right) \end{array} \right] \tag{3}$$

4.1. Handling Exception Propagation

In section 2, the problem of exception propagation was discussed. Figure 3 shows a simple diagram of a frame which raises an exception, but has no local handler for that exception:

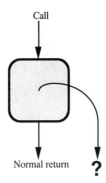

Figure 3

In this case, we see that the frame has a single entry point, but two possible exit points (the normal exit and the exception propagation). If the exception is being propagated across a subprogram call, then we cannot statically determine its target handler. This leads us to the following conclusion:

- When an exception can be propagated out of a frame, the worst case execution time of that frame in isolation cannot be determined statically.

This conclusion implies that exceptions can only be analysed if the calling frames of all exception-propagating frames are also available for analysis. In summary:

- To determine WCET for a frame in isolation, it must have a single entry and a single exit point. This means that a frame can only be analysed for WCET if no exceptions can propagate from it. Formally, for a frame **i** to be analysable in isolation, we require that:

$$(RAISED(i) \cup LEBOT(i)) - HANDLED(i) = \varnothing \tag{4}$$

- In general, exceptions and their propagation can only be analysed if all the compilation units forming a task body or the main program are available simultaneously for analysis. In the worst-case, this means that all timing analysis must be deferred until the program's linking phase. Program unit bodies that are not available could be analysed by requiring that weak-propagation annotations are placed in their specifications.

- If an unhandled exception can propagate to the outermost scope of a task body or the main program, then timing analysis is infeasible. This is unsurprising as it means that a program may terminate in an uncontrolled manner at run-time.

As an example, consider the following diagram which shows a subprogram call between two frames, the latter of which can raise an exception. The outer frame has a handler for that exception, allowing the timing properties of that frame to be resolved:

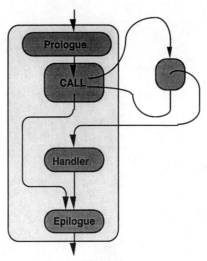

Figure 4

To analyse the timing behaviour of this frame, we must not only consider the exceptions that may be raised in the code of the frame itself, but also in the declarative parts or statements of any other frames that are called. Equation 3 given above for WCET(frame) is therefore no longer sufficient - the set of exceptions that can possibly be propagated into a frame "from below" must also be considered. Exception flow analysis can supply this information. In addition to the RAISED set, the live-exceptions set LEBOT must be considered. The equation for WCET(frame) is modified thus:

$$WCET(frame) = WCET(prologue) + WCET(epilogue) +$$

$$\max \begin{bmatrix} WCET(code) \\ \max_{\forall E: E \subseteq (LEBOT \cup RAISED)} \begin{pmatrix} WCET(code) + WCPT + \\ {}_{raise\,E} \\ WCFINDT + WCET(handler) \\ {}_{E\_ID=E} \end{pmatrix} \end{bmatrix} \quad (5)$$

For exceptions that are propagated into a frame, the notation:

$$WCET(code)_{raise\,E}$$

now refers to the WCET for the code of the frame *including* the code of any called frames up to the point where the exception E is raised. This model is still not entirely accurate - it does not consider the time required to propagate the exception. The time taken to do this is proportional to the number of times an exception is propagated before a handler is found. Some further new notation is therefore required:

WCHFT	The worst case time for a handler to *fail* to find a handler for the current exception.
N_E	The number of times the exception under consideration is propagated before a handler is successfully found.

The value of WCHFT is basically the time needed for each handler in the dynamic call chain to evaluate all the if/elsif parts and conclude that no handler for the current exception can be found. With the compiled-handlers approach, WCHFT is different for each frame because each frame potentially has a different number of handlers. With the static-tables approach WCHFT is constant since the global exception table is of constant size and hence any unsuccessful search through it will take constant time. Incorporating these values into our equation for WCET(frame) gives:

$$WCET(frame) = WCET(prologue) + WCET(epilogue) +$$

$$\max \begin{bmatrix} WCET(code) \\ \\ \max_{\forall E:E\subseteq(LEBOT\cup RAISED)} \begin{pmatrix} WCET(code) + WCPT + \\ \text{\scriptsize raise E} \\ (N_E \times WCHFT) + WCFINDT + \\ WCET(handler) \\ \text{\scriptsize E\_ID=E} \end{pmatrix} \end{bmatrix} \quad (6)$$

Note that if ($N_E = 0$) and (LEBOT = $\emptyset$) are substituted into equation 6 (i.e. when no exceptions are propagated into the frame, and all other exceptions are handled locally), then this reduces to equation 3 given above.

4.2 Timing analysis method

We now have enough information to develop a method for the analysis of the worst case timing of a program written in our subset. We assume that a method for determining the WCET of normal code sequences, handlers, and the relevant parts of the runtime system already exists[5].

Essentially the analysis proceeds as follows:

1) Build the control-flow and context graphs for the entire program or task body.
2) For each frame, determine
   - i)   The RAISED set.
   - ii) The HANDLED set.
   - iii) The $WCET(code)$, $WCET(code)$, and $WCET(handler)$ for each exception E
          $\text{\scriptsize raise E} \quad \text{\scriptsize E\_ID=E}$
          in the frame.
3) Using exception flow analysis, determine LEBOT for each frame.
4) Check that no exceptions can be propagated from the main program using equation 4.
5) From LEBOT, trace the flow of exception propagation and determine N_E for each exception in each frame.
6) Apply equation 6 to determine WCET(frame) for each frame that has handlers.
7) Determine WCET for the entire program or task body by composing the WCETs for each constituent frame.

We assume the values of WCPT, WCHFT and WCFINDT are known, although they will, of course, be both compiler- and target-dependent.

4.3 An example

Consider the following program.

```
procedure A is
   procedure B is
      procedure C is
```

```
      begin
        -- statements that might
        -- raise CONSTRAINT_ERROR
       end C;
      begin
       C;
      end B;

      procedure D is
      begin
        -- statements that might
        -- raise STORAGE_ERROR;
       end D;

     begin
       B;
       D;
     exception
       when CONSTRAINT_ERROR =>
       -- handlers
       when STORAGE_ERROR =>
       -- ...
     end A;
```

The context graph for this program is shown in figure 5. The start context S (representing the Ada environment task) has been added.

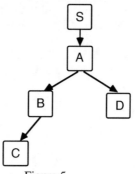

Figure 5

Exception flow analysis yields RAISED, HANDLED, and LEBOT as shown in table 1.

We can now apply our test from equation 4 to see which contexts are analysable. Only contexts A and S pass the test. S represents the main environment task, so we may conclude that the whole program is analysable. The context graph is then searched bottom-up to determine how many times each exception may be propagated.

Context	RAISED	HANDLED	LEBOT
S	∅	∅	∅
A	∅	STORAGE_ERROR CONSTRAINT_ERROR	STORAGE_ERROR CONSTRAINT_ERROR
B	∅	∅	CONSTRAINT_ERROR
C	CONSTRAINT_ERROR	∅	∅
D	STORAGE_ERROR	∅	∅

Table 1

For instance, the CONSTRAINT_ERROR raised in C appears twice in the LEBOT sets for B and A before disappearing in S. This means N_E is 2 for that particular occurrence of CONSTRAINT-ERROR. Similarly, we discover that STORAGE _ERROR raised in D can only be propagated once before being handled. The worst case time for procedure A can then be determined by applying equation 6.

5. Conclusions and further work

This paper has presented a detailed review of the features and implementation of exception handling in Ada83. Through this study, a model for the static timing analysis of exceptions has been developed. We feel this model is general enough to be applied to most implementations of Ada.

The York Ada compilation system[11] is currently supported by a prototype worst-case execution time tool[5]. The compilation system and timing tool target a bare 68020-based microcomputer. The timing tool supports our language subset but does not attempt any form of exception flow analysis, relying on purely syntactic means. Its analysis is therefore rather pessimistic when exceptions are used. In the near future we plan to introduce weak-propagation annotations to the analysed language. This will be followed by improving the tool to support exception flow analysis. These improvements will be complemented by a symbolic execution tool that will perform inter-procedural constant-propagation, dead-code elimination and so on. This tool will also be able to produce verification conditions in the style of the SPARK examiner[12]. It is possible that the use of weak propagation annotations will allow verification condition generation to be performed for both the normal and exception paths of a program.

Finally, we plan to introduce some features of Ada9X into our subset, including a limited form of tasking and protected objects. Non-nested, library-level tasks and protected objects will be allowed supported by certain features of the Ada9X real-time systems annex, notably priority ceiling inheritance scheduling. Our model for exception analysis is largely unchanged by these additions. Recent advances in schedulability analysis[13] will allow the construction of large parallel systems with totally predictable timing properties.

Acknowledgements

The authors thank Peter Fenelon and John McDermid for their valuable comments on an early draft of this paper. This work has been wholly funded by British Aerospace PLC through the Dependable Computing Systems Centre at the Univeristy of York.

References

[1]   Park, C.Y., *Predicting Program Execution Times by Analyzing Static and Dynamic Program Paths.* Journal of Real-Time Systems, 1993. **5**: p. 31-62.

[2]   Pospischil, G., *et al.*, *Developing Real-Time Tasks with Predictable Performance.* IEEE Software, 1992. **9**: p. 35-44.

[3]   Stoyenko, A.D., C. Hamacher, and R.C. Holt, *Analyzing Hard Real-Time Programs for Guaranteed Schedulability.* IEEE Transactions on Software Engineering, 1991. **17**(8): p. 737-750.

[4]   Baker, T.P. and G.A. Riccardi, *Implementing Ada Exceptions*. IEEE Software, 1986. **3**(5): p.
        43-51.

[5]   Forsyth, C.H., *Implementation of the Worst-Case Execution Time Analyser*. June 1992, York
        Software Engineering Ltd., University of York: Task 8 Volume E Deliverable on ESTEC
        contract 9198/90/NL/SF

[6]   Carre, B.A., *et al.*, *SPARK: the SPADE Ada Kernel (edition 3.1)*. 1992, Program Validation
        Ltd.

[7]   Winterstein, D. and R. Holzapfel, *The Use of Ada for Safety Critical Applications: Appendix
        A: Safe Ada Language Study*. 1987, EuroFighter/Systeam.

[8]   Luckham, D.C., *et al.*, *ANNA: A language for annotating Ada programs*. Lecture notes in
        Computer Science, ed. G. Goos and J. Hartmanis. Vol. 260. 1987, Springer-Verlag. 143.

[9]   Baker, D.A. and S.M. Sutton, *Exception Flow Analysis in Ada*. 1986, Department of
        Computer Science, University of Colorado, Boulder.

[10]   Sutton, S.M., *Personal communication*. 1992,

[11]   Firth, J.R., C.H. Forsyth, and I.C. Wand, *York Ada Compiler Release 4 User Guide*. 1989,
        Department of Computer Science, University of York.

[12]   Carré, B., J. Garnsworthy, and W. Marsh. *SPARK - A Safety-Related Ada Subset*. in *AdaUK
        1992*. 1992. London, U.K.: IOS Press.

[13]   Audsley, N., *et al.*, *Applying New Scheduling Theory to Static Priority Pre-emptive
        Scheduling*. Software Engineering Journal, 1993. **to appear**.

Ada: Towards Maturity
Ed. L. Collingbourne
IOS Press 1993

Text Formatting facilities for Ada

John Smart

BAeSema, Biwater House, Portsmouth Road, Esher, Surrey, KT10 9SJ.

Abstract. This paper describes an Ada package that provides text formatting facilities which have been derived from the mechanisms used by the languages C, Algol 68 and C++. The package combines the flexibility and ease of use of format control strings with the type-safety inherent in Ada so that values of any data type, including types defined by the user, can be conveniently and safely converted into their textual form within a piece of formatted text. The textual form may be retained in memory, for later use, or written to an Ada Text_Io file. These formatting facilities have also been extended to provide user control over the formatting of values of the types *Calendar.Time* and *Calendar.Duration* which are based on the ANSI C format controls for *strftime*. The paper concludes by discussing some of the Ada 83 implementation issues that arose from the desire to achieve an efficient implementation of interfaces that are simple to use and indicates that Ada 9X should overcome such problems.

1. Introduction

The facilities of Ada's built in Text_Io package are quite inconvenient and verbose to use as the means to produce consistently tabulated textual output from an Ada program that contains many different data types. By the time the necessary Text_Io generics have been instantiated for the base types and the logic has been written to maintain columnar layout one finds that at least a page of Ada source has been produced where the logical connections between the statements are not obvious. If the textual layout needs to be changed one is faced with a significant source code modification task with its attendant recompilation, linking and testing overheads.

In contrast, the `printf()` interface of C is easy and concise to use but is not type safe, in that the types of the values to be converted into text are deduced from the format control patterns given by the formatting string. Algol 68 provided Formatted Transput composed of a format denotation associated with a value-list of mixed types which could be scalar or aggregates. In this case, however, the translation is type-safe in that the types of the values in the value-list determined how the format denotation was interpreted. The C++ iostream class library has abandoned the use of a formatting string in favour of overloaded operators which exploit the fact that all classes can know how to translate themselves into text and can therefore provide their own version of the overloaded operator. This is notationally expressive and concise until one needs to control the format using manipulators when the output expressions can become long-winded and repetitive.

The objectives in developing the Formatting_Text package for Ada were to combine the conciseness, type-safety and extensibility of overloading an operator with the expressiveness of format denotations to specify the layout required. The rest of this section outlines the basic operations provided by the package and the mechanisms that ensure it is type-safe in use.

The second section gives a full description of the notation used within the formatting string to translate values of basic types and to control their layout in the generated text. The third section describes the generic interfaces that allow the same facilities to be extended to any derived or user-defined types. The fourth and fifth sections show how the facilities can also be used to direct the formatted text into any Text_Io file or a memory resident structure. The sixth section describes how the same mechanisms have been applied to the built-in types, Calendar.Time and Calendar.Duration, to give the user straightforward control over their formatting. The final section describes several different implementation strategies that were considered and rejected in favour of strategies that ensured efficiency at run time and which simplified the use of the interfaces. Unfortunately these strategies are not entirely in keeping with the style of Ada 83, although it appears that they will be accommodated by Ada 9X.

1.1. Overview of the basic operations

The interfaces of the package, **Formatting_Text**, utilise a formatting string to specify the text pattern into which data values of any type are to be mapped and to control the textual representation of values of all basic types. The package utilises the facilities of Ada's **Text_Io** package to convert the basic data types into human-readable form. Any user-defined data type can also be mapped into a formatting string once the appropriate generic function from the **Formatting_Text** package has been instantiated for the type. The basic features which are described in this section utilise the declarations shown in Table 1 which are taken from the specification of the **Formatting_Text** package.

To produce a formatted string the parameter to the **Put** or **Put_Line** procedures has to be an expression that delivers a value of the type **Formatter**. The **stdout** or **cout** functions have to be used as the left-most argument of this expression since they are the only operations that generate a value of the **limited private** type **Formatter** from a standard Ada type; the overloaded **"and"** operators.will then propogate this type through to the end of the expression evaluation.

Table 1.   The basic declarations of the Formatting_Text package

```
type Format_Integer is range System.MIN_INT ..  System.MAX_INT;
type Format_Float    is digits System.MAX_DIGITS;
      subtype Int  is Format_Integer;
      subtype Real is Format_Float;
type Formatter       is limited private;
function Stdout (Format : String) return Formatter;
function Cout    (Format : String) return Formatter;
function Stdout return Formatter;
function Cout    return Formatter;
function "and" (L : Formatter; R : Boolean)          return Formatter;
function "and" (L : Formatter; R : Character)         return Formatter;
function "and" (L : Formatter; R : String)            return Formatter;
function "and" (L : Formatter; R : Format_Integer) return Formatter;
function "and" (L : Formatter; R : Format_Float)     return Formatter;
function "and" (L : Formatter; R : System.Address) return Formatter;
function "<=" (L : Formatter; Defaults : String)     return Formatter;
procedure Put        (P : Formatter);
procedure Put_Line (P : Formatter);
```

The `stdout` function is used to direct the constructed string onto Ada's `Standard_Output` file whilst the `cout` function is used to direct the constructed string onto Ada's `Current_Output` file. The `Put` and `Put_Line` procedures simply ensure that the complete formatted string is delivered to the specified file, with a subsequent New_Line in the case of the `Put_Line` procedure.

Thus, the statement: `Put_Line(Stdout and "Hello World");` will write the string `Hello World` to Ada's `Standard_Output` file and follow it with a `Text_Io.New_Line` operation. On the other hand, the statement: `Put_Line(Cout and "Hello World");` will write the string `Hello World` to Ada's `current_output` file and follow it with a `Text_Io.New_Line` operation. If, however, the `current_output` file is closed then the string will be automatically redirected into the `standard_Output` file. This ensures that the string is always output, even if the file into which `current_output` has been redirected by a `Text_Io.Set_Output` operation is closed before another `Text_Io.Set_Output` operation is performed.

As well as handling strings the interface can format numeric values (type converted to `Int` or `Real`), booleans, characters and System.Address. Type conversion of numeric values can be avoided by instantiating the generics described in section 3.

Straightforward formatting can be achieved by use of the parameterless versions of `Stdout` and `cout`, thus: `Put_Line(Cout and "x =" and Int(x) and "y =" and Real(y));` will produce, for example: `x = 1234 y = 56.788999` since each value formatted is automatically followed by a space character. To produce more sophisticated formatting the versions of `stdout` and `cout` that take a string parameter have to be used.

The parameter of the `stdout` or `cout` functions must be a `string` value (either a literal or the value of a string variable). This string is used to control, in the fashion described below, the conversion and formatting of the values supplied as the right hand arguments of the `"and"` functions. These `"and"` functions can only operate on values of the `limited private` type `Formatter`. The versions of the `stdout` or `cout` functions which are parameterless assume that the use of a standard string, as described at the end of this section.

The left hand argument of the `"and"` functions must be a value of the `limited private` type `Formatter` which can only be produced by the `stdout`, `cout` or another `"and"` function. This strong type control ensures that the facilities cannot be misused and that the `"and"` functions are always evaluated from left to right. The strong typing also ensures that the right hand arguments of the `"and"` functions are always correctly converted into their textual representation.

These `"and"` functions are used to construct a 'text formatting' expression, the result of which can also be written to any Ada `Text_Io.File_Type` or the user-accessible data type, `Text_Buffer_T`, defined by the package. These additional destinations for a formatted text string are described in sections 4 and 5. For simplicity, the description, and examples, of the text formatting features of the package are given in terms of delivering the result to the `Current_Output` file.

1.2. Text formatting expression evaluation

A 'text formatting' expression always takes the form:

```
Destination_Function (Formatting_String) [and value]
```

and these expressions can only be used as the parameter of the `Put` or `Put_Line` procedures, for the reason given above.

The use of an Ada expression allows any number of data values to be formatted into a formatted text string in a single Ada statement and provides a concise and efficient notation

Table 2. Simple examples of formatting text

```
declare
      x   : Format_Integer := 1234;
      y   : Format_Float   :=    56.789;
      z   : Boolean := True;
begin
      Put_Line (Cout ("&s ") and x and y and z);
      Put_Line (Cout ("x = &s, y = &s, z = &s")       and x and y and z);
      Put_Line (Cout ("x = &s && y = &s && z = &s") and x and y and z);
end;
-------- Will generate the following text: -------
      1234 56.788999 TRUE
      x = 1234, y = 56.788999, z = TRUE
      x = 1234 & y = 56.788999 & z = TRUE
```

for the construction of formatted text. The "**and**" operator has been overloaded because it is one of the set of operators with the lowest precedence in Ada; its use minimises the need to use parentheses to control precedence within these expressions.

It should be noted, from Table 1, that the types **Format_Integer** and **Format_Float** have been specified to have the largest integer and float range supported by an Ada implementation. Values of smaller integer and float types, as well as any fixed type, can be used by type converting them into either of these two types; the subtypes **Int** and **Real** have been provided for such type conversions. Section 3.2 describes how values of smaller discrete and real data types can be directly used in formatting expressions. The simplest ways of formatting values of these types, with the facilities of the **Formatting_Text** package, are shown in Table 2.

From the above it can be seen that a value that follows an "**and**" operator is translated and injected into the generated formatted string wherever the formatting string contains a '**&**' character. The '**&**' character has been used, in preference to the '**%**' character used in C, because of its general use as a catenation operator in Ada. To produce an '**&**' character in the generated text two consecutive **&**'s must occur in the formatting string.

It is the right-hand values of the "**and**" functions which trigger the interpretation of the formatting string. For each value encountered, the characters of the formatting string are copied into a Formatting Buffer until the control character '**&**' is found. The character pattern after the '**&**' is used to control the translation and formatting of the value into the generated text at the point reached. This generation of text characters from a text formatting expression is shown in Figure 1.

If, during the search for a '**&**' character, the end of the formatting string is reached then the interpretation continues from the beginning of the formatting string; this repetitive interpretation of the formatting string will continue until all the values to be formatted have been processed. If the formatting string contains no '**&**' characters it is only copied into the generated text once, when the first value is processed; any other values are simply appended to this text with a default translation into a textual form.

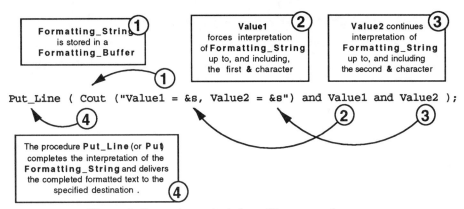

Figure 1. Processing a text formatting expression

This ensures that every value that appears as the right-hand value of an "**and**" function is always translated into the generated text. Thus, the statement: `Put_Line (Cout ("Values are: ") and x and z and y);` produces, `Values are: 1234TRUE56.788999`

To ensure that each formatted value is separated from its neighbour it can be expressed as: `Put_Line (Cout ("&s ") and "Values are:" and x and z and y);` to produce: `Values are: 1234 TRUE 56.788999`

The parameterless version of `stdout` and `cout` functions automatically apply the standard formatting string "`&s `" to the values supplied so that this common situation can be written more concisely as: `Put_Line (Cout and "Values are:" and x and z and y);`

If there are insufficient "**and**" functions to match the complete formatting string, the uninterpreted part of the formatting string is appended to the generated text, with any remaining formatting patterns removed, so that: `Put_Line (Cout ("x = &s, y = &s, z = &s") and x and y);` produces: `x = 1234, y = 56.788999, z =`

2. The formatting control facilities

2.1. Conversion of values into text

Each '`&`' character in the formatting string acts as a placeholder in the generated text for the value which will replace it. The characters following a '`&`' character constitute a formatting control pattern which determines how the value will be translated and formatted. A format control pattern is always terminated by a character which determines the mode of translation that is to be applied to a value, as defined in Table 3.

Ada's strong typing ensures that the type of each value to be formatted is known to be either:

- an integer, (including a System.Address)
  - a real,
  - or a string (which may be an enumeration literal).

This knowledge is used to apply the default translation of a value into its textual form when the format control character does not supply a translation mode for the type of value encountered.

Table 3. Translation Mode characters in a Format Control Pattern

Type of Value	Mode Character	Interpretation	Example - with default justification
Integer (e.g.27)	s (default)	Decimal value	27
	b	Binary value	11011
	B	Ada binary literal	2#11011#
	o	Octal value	33
	O	Ada octal literal	8#33#
	d	Decimal value	27
	x	Hexadecimal value	1B
	X	Ada hexadecimal value	16#1B#
Real (e.g. 12.34)	s (default)	Fixed Point notation	12.339999
	e	Exponential notation	1.239999E+1
	f	Fixed point notation	12.339999
String or Enumeration (e.g. A Text_piece)	s (default)	as is (enumeration in Uppercase)	A Text_piece
	U	Uppercase	A TEXT_PIECE
	L	Lowercase	a text_piece
	E	European case[1]	A Text_Piece
	any other character	as the default character s for the type of value	

These formatting facilities can be easily used to generate formatted strings which are very sensitive to their context, for example:

```
declare Suffix : array (Boolean) of String (1..4) := ("ices", "ex   ");
begin   Put_Line (Cout ("&s ind&s found.") and x and Suffix (x = 1));
```

will produce:

```
10 indices found.  -- when x = 10
1 index   found.        -- when x = 1
```

2.2. Controlling the layout of values

The above examples show that, by default, the translation of the right-hand values of the "and" functions always generates the smallest number of characters needed to represent the value; no padding characters are added.

2.2.1. Controlling a value field

The user can control the layout of the generated text by specifying: 1) the field width for a value, 2) the justification of a value within its field, 3) the precision of real values, and 4) the character to be used to pad a translated value to a specified field width

These layout controls must appear between the '&' character and the translation mode character in the order listed in Table 4.

---

[1] European case is interpreted as follows: the first character of a word, and characters immediately preceded by an underscore, '_' are converted into Upper case; all other characters are converted to lower case.

Table 4.   Layout control notation and order

Layout Control	Value	Interpretation	Default (when absent)
W - field width	integer	Width of field	Exact width of value
J - justification	character:	Justification of the string within the specified field:	
	.	Default (to separate **W** value from **P** value)	Left justification for text, Right justification for numbers
	>	Right	
	<	Left	
	I	Centre	
P - precision	integer	Number of places after the decimal point	6
F - filling	_ c	Use the character **c** as the field filler character	' ' (blank)

Another important characteristic of the interface is that any strings, or data values that have been converted to strings, can never be truncated during formatting as a result of specifying a field width that is not wide enough.

Each of the layout controls is optional but if present, they must be specified in the order WJPF, shown by Table 4. The layout control facilities can be used to simplify the production of neatly tabulated text, thus:

```
Put_Line (Cout ("&13e ") and x and y and z);
-- produces:                     1234    5.678899E+1 TRUE
Put_Line (Cout ("&13_.X ") and x and y and z);
-- produces:             ......16#1D2# ....56.788999 TRUE........
Put_Line (Cout ("&13>3__L ") and x and y and z);
-- produces:             _____1234 _____56.789 _____true
```

2.2.2. Repeated formatting substrings

Obviously the automatic repetition of a formatting string, as shown above, will not give the desired result if one wishes to precede or follow the repeated sequence with some other text. For example, the statement:

```
Put_Line (Cout ("Values:&8.3f produced") and x and y and z);
```

will produce:

```
Values:    1234 producedValues:   56.789 producedValues:TRUE        produced
```

To allow the desired format to be generated in these cases the format control pattern can specify that substrings are to be repeated by the use of the characters { and } to delimit the substring. For example:

```
Put_Line (Cout ("Values:&3{&8>3f} produced") and x and y and z);
```

will produce:

```
Values:    1234   56.789      TRUE produced
```

The number of repetitions is specified between the & and the opening { character. The repetition of the enclosed substring is automatically terminated as soon as there are no further values in the expression, that is, when there are fewer "**and**" operations than given by the repetition count. The repetition control mechanism cannot be nested inside another one.

2.2.3. Controlling the default translations

Circumstances can arise where it is necessary to change the default translations for more than one type of value within a formatting expression. For example, one may require all integer values to be translated into hexadecimal, all real values to be exponential and all string values to be in lower case. This could be achieved by providing an explicit control pattern for each value, thus:

```
Put_Line (Cout ("&10_.X&10.3_,e &10_.L") and x and y and z);
```
will print:

```
...16#1D2#..5.679E+1 true......
```

This, however, requires that the formatting string is expanded to explicitly control the translation of each value. The overloaded operator "<=" has been provided to allow the default translation of values to be changed for the subsequent interpretation of the values to be formatted within a single formatting expression. The right hand argument of the "<=" function is a formatting string which is interpreted as specifying the new default values of the Mode, Justification and Precision for the rest of the expression. Thus:

```
Put_Line (Cout ("&10_.s") <= "&X&.3e&>L" and x and y and z and z and x);
```
will print:

```
...16#1D2#..5.679E+1......true......true...16#1D2#
```
because the string after the "<=" sets the Integer Mode to x, the Real Precision to 3 and the String Mode to L and its Justification to > (Right Justification); whilst the Formatting String simply specifies that all values are to use a Field Width of 10 and the Fill Character of . (dot).

2.3. Position control

The spacing between formatted values can also be controlled by use of the position control notation which is expressed as &Np where the integer value N defines the position in the formatting buffer (starting at 1), of the next character to be inserted. If the buffer position N has already been filled then the notation &Np has no effect. For example:

```
Put_Line (Cout ("&8pValues:&3{&8>3f}&45 .pproduced") and x and y and z);
                (^ position at 8)   (^ fill to position 45 with .)
```
will produce:

```
        Values:    1234  56.789       TRUE......produced
   Column ^8                                    ^45
```

2.4. Injecting New_Line operations

The formatting notation also allows Text_Io.New_Line operations to be injected into the generated text by use of the notation &Nn, where the optional integer value N specifies the number of consecutive Text_Io.New_Line operations to be applied. For example:

```
Put_Line(Cout("Values:&2n&3{&16>3f&n}&nproduced.") and x and y and z);
will produce:
Values:
```

```
        1234
        56.789
          TRUE
```

```
produced.
```

This effect is achieved by flushing the characters, that are currently in the formatting buffer, onto the specified output file so that the operation **Text_Io.New_Line** can be called with appropriate parameters at the required point. This avoids having to represent a New_Line operation within the generated character string. It also has the beneficial side effect of effectively removing any limit on the number of characters that can be generated from a single formatting statement so long as a single line of output does not exceed the size of the formatting buffer used internally by the **Formatting_Text** package. This buffer has a size of 128 characters.

3. Support for derived types

In the specification of the package, **Formatting_Text**, the routines described above are supplemented by eight generic functions which support the formatting of all other derived and user-defined types. The full specification of these generics is given in Table 5. and their use is described in this Section. As always, these generics should only be instantiated, for specific actual parameters, once per program if at all possible. One way to ensure this is to include the instantiations in the packages which declare the types they use; an effective Ada compiler will not bind them into a program image if they are not called.

Table 5. The generic functions for formatting user-defined types

```
generic                type Enum_Type    is (<>);
function And_Enum      (L : Formatter; R : Enum_Type)       return Formatter;

generic                type Fixed_Type   is delta <>;
function And_Fixed     (L : Formatter; R : Fixed_Type)      return Formatter;

generic                type Integer_Type is range <>;
function And_Integer (L : Formatter; R : Integer_Type) return Formatter;

generic                type Float_Type   is digits <>;
function And_Float     (L : Formatter; R : Float_Type)      return Formatter;

generic                type A_Type         is limited private;
                       type Access_Type  is access A_Type;
function And_Access    (L : Formatter; R : Access_Type)     return Formatter;

generic                type User_Type      is limited private;
with function Formatting_Function (Into : Formatting_Buffer;
                                   This : User_Type)        return Formatter;
function And_User_Type(L : Formatter; R : User_Type)        return Formatter;

generic   type an_Element is private;
          type Index_Type is (<>);
          type Array_Type is Array (Index_Type range <>) of an_Element;
     with function And_Element
               (L : Formatter; R : an_Element)         return Formatter;
function And_Array (L : Formatter; R : Array_Type)         return Formatter;

generic   type an_Element is private;
          type Index_Type is (<>);
          type Array_Type is Array (Index_Type) of an_Element;
     with function And_Element (L : Formatter;
                                R : an_Element)         return Formatter;
function And_Bound_Array    (L : Formatter;
                             R : Array_Type)            return Formatter;
```

On the other hand, the bodies of these generics are so short that they have been subject to **Pragma Inline** statements so that the function bodies are replaced by inline code; they could then be instantiated locally as often as needed without introducing any runtime overhead.

3.1. Enumeration types

The generic function **And_Enum** enables the user to define an "**and**" function for an enumeration type which can then be used in the same way as the "**and**" function for the type **Boolean**, thus:

```
type My_Enum is (Repair, Slice);
function "and" is new And_Enum (My_Enum );
Enum_Object : My_Enum := Repair ;
```

This operator can now be invoked in the same way as in the examples above:

```
Put_Line (Cout ("The &s is done.") and Enum_Object);
```

will print: **The REPAIR is done.**

The same formatted string will be produced by:

```
Put_Line (Cout ("The &s is done." and My_Enum'Image (Enum_Object));
```

but the generated code is larger and slower than the former statement due to the fact that **'Image** returns an unconstrained string. However, each instantiation of the generic function, **And_Enum**, will itself instantiate **Text_Io.Enum_Io** to allow the enumeration type values to be converted into a string. The overhead of instantiating **And_Enum** is only worthwhile if the instantiated function is used several times. It should be noted that either approach will cause a table of the enumeration literal values to be built into the program's image.

3.2. Types derived from the built-in types

In the same way that **And_Enum** has been instantiated above for an enumeration type the generic functions **And_Fixed**, **And_Float** and **And_Integer** can be instantiated for any Fixed, Float or Integer type respectively to provide special "**and**" functions for such data types.

These functions simply type convert their parameter into a **Format_Float**, or a **Format_Integer**. These same conversions could simply be applied explicitly to values of any numeric type as shown in Table 6.

Obviously the use of the instantiated functions produces more concise, readable and type-safe source code but it generates calls to the instantiated functions to achieve the type conversions producing a small run time overhead. Explicit type conversions produce more verbose source code and achieves the type conversions inline at the cost of generating more code on each use. It is therefore probably only worthwhile to instantiate these generics if there are many instances of their use in which case they should be instantiated as part of the data type declarations.

3.3. Support for other user types

The generic function **And_User_Type**, shown in Table 5, enables the user to create an "**and**" function for any user defined type for which the formatted text is more complex than that produced by a basic type. To instantiate this generic function the user must have implemented the function, which will be supplied as an actual parameter to the instantiation.

Table 6. Using instantiations of the numeric formatting generics

```
type Metres_Type  is new Float;
type Bearing_Type is range 0 .. 65535;
type F16_8_T is delta  2.0**(-8) range -2.0**7 .. 2.0**7 - 2.0**(-8);
function "and" is new And_Float   (Metres_Type);
function "and" is new And_Integer (Bearing_Type);
function "and" is new And_Fixed   (F16_8_T);
Distance : Metres_Type  :=   1000.25;
Angle    : Bearing_Type := 12_500;
Value    : F16_8_T      :=     99.9;
begin
    Put_Line (Cout (" &s") and Distance and Value and Angle);
    Put_Line (Cout (" &s") and Real (Distance)
                           and Real (Value)
                           and Int  (Angle));
end;  -- will produce:
    1000.249999 99.899999 125000
    1000.249999 99.899999 125000
```

This user written function must format a value of the user type into another **limited private** type, **Formatting_Buffer**, by using any of the **"and"** functions which are available in conjunction with the **Format** function provided by the **Formatting_Text** package with the following specification:

```
type Formatting_Buffer is limited private;
function Format(L: Formatting_Buffer; Format: string) return Formatter;
```

Table 7. Instantiating and using a formatting function for a user-defined typed

```
type Cartesian_Position_T is record
    X_Coordinate: Float;
    Y_Coordinate: Float;
end record;
function Format_Cartesian_Posn (
                Into : Formatting_Buffer,
                From : Cartesian_Position_T) return Formatter is
 begin
     return Format (Into, "(x=&5.2_0f, y=&5.2_0f)")
                          and Real (From.X_Coordinate)
                          and Real (From.Y_Coordinate);
 end Format_Cartesian_Posn;
function "and" is new
    And_User_Type(User_Type        => Cartesian_Position_T,
                  Format_User_Type => Format_Cartesian_Posn);
-- The user can now format strings containing text representations of this data type, thus:
Posn1 : Cartesian_Position_T := ( 60.0,    55.5);
Posn2 : Cartesian_Position_T := (  1.123,   6.6);
begin
Put_Line (Cout ("Positions are&20>_.s&20>_.s") and Posn1 and Posn2);
-- will print:
Positions are....(x=60.00, y=55.50)....(x=01.12, y=06.60)
```

An example of creating and using an **"and"** function for a user-defined type is given in Table 7.

Note that the formatted text of the user type produced by the instantiated "and" function is treated as a string value when it is used and can be justified and manipulated just like any other string value, so:

Put_Line (Cout ("Positions are &U, &U") and Posn1 and Posn2);
will print:

Positions are (X=60.00, Y=55.50), (X=01.12, Y=06.60)

3.4. Array types

The above facilities allow single values of any type to be included in a formatting expression. Arrays of values can only be formatted with the above facilities by writing a specific formatting procedure for each size, and type, of array required. This is time consuming, error prone and produces formatted strings that cannot be used in a formatting expression.

The **Formatting_Text** package therefore provides the generic functions, **And_Array** and **And_Bound_Array** shown in Table 6, that can be instantiated for any unconstrained or constrained array type respectively. Two generics are provided to accommodate Ada's constraint that a generic formal array type and the actual array subtype must be either both constrained or unconstrained

The formal generic function specifies the formatting function to be used to format an element of the array. Once these generics have been instantiated, values of the array type can be included in a formatting expression just like a value of a basic type. The instantiated function keeps track of the number of array elements to be formatted so that each array element value causes the next pattern in the format control string to be interpreted.

An example of instantiating and using an "and" function for an array type is shown in Table 8.

Table 8. Instantiating and using a formatting function for an array type

```
     type Int_List is array (positive range <>) of Integer;
I_List : Int_List (1..23) := (
              -99, -89, -79, -69, -59, -49, -39, -29, -19, 9,
               99,  89,  79,  69,  59,  49,  39,  29,  19, 9, 1, 2, 3);
function "and"         is new And_Integer (Integer);
function And_Int_List is new And_Array (an_Element => Integer,
                                         Index_Type  => positive,
                                         Array_Type  => Int_List,
                                         And_Element => "and");
function "and" (L : Formatter; R : Int_List) return Formatter
                renames And_Int_List;
Put_Line (Cout ("Array:&n&8p&6{&5s&5s&5s&5s&5s&n}&nValues") and I_List;
-- will print:
Array:
          -99  -89  -79  -69  -59
          -49  -39  -29  -19   -9
           99   89   79   69   59
           49   39   29   19    9
            1    2    3
Values
```

Note that the `And_Integer` generic has had to be instantiated for the `Integer` element type since the elements cannot be subjected to an explicit type conversion and that the operator "`and`" has to be defined by a `renames` when the And_Element function is itself an "`and`" operator.

3.4.1. Iterating over array elements

This is reasonably expressive except for the fact that the repetition count has a hard coded integer value specified (`&6{...}` in the above statement) which requires the user to anticipate the probable size of the array being formatted. To overcome this problem the repetition count can be specified as the * character which is interpreted to mean: 'until all array elements have been processed'. This makes it possible to write formatting expressions which will work correctly with any size of array, thus:

```
Put_Line (Cout ("I_List (&s ,, &s):&n&*{&8p&5s&5s&5s&5s&5s&n}&n")
                and I_List'First and I_List'Last and I_List;
```

will print:

```
I_List (1 .. 23):
        -99  -89  -79  -69  -59
        -49  -39  -29  -19   -9
         99   89   79   69   59
         49   39   29   19    9
          1    2    3
```

3.4.2. Boolean array example

The above approach could be used to format an array of Booleans, but this would produce the enumeration literal value, `TRUE` or `FALSE`, for each element in the Boolean array. A more concise representation of a Boolean array could be produced by instantiating the generic function, `And_User_Type` for such arrays as shown in Table 9.

With this "`and`" function for the `Flags` array type, the following block statement:

Table 9. Defining a formatter for Boolean Arrays

```
type Flags is array (Positive range <>) of Boolean;
     Pragma Pack (Flags);
function Format_Flags (Into : Formatting_Buffer;
                       From : Flags)                      return Formatter is
        -- define a function to convert a Boolean value to '0' or '1'
    function Format_Bool (Into : Formatter;
                          From : Boolean)                 return Formatter is
      Bit : constant array (Boolean) of Character := ('0', '1');
    begin
          return Into and Bit (From);
    end Format_Bool;
                 -- instantiate a Boolean Array formatter using Format_Bool as the element formatter
    function "and" is new
                      And_Array (Boolean, Positive, Flags, Format_Bool);
begin    -- convert Flags into a string of '0's and '1's
      return Format (Into, "&*{&s}") and From;
end Format_Flags;
function "and" is new And_User_Type (Flags, Format_Flags);
```

```
declare
  My_Flags : Flags(1..12) := ( True,    True,    True, False, False, False,
                                True, False, False,    True, False,    True);
begin
  Put_Line (Cout ("My_Flags are &s;") and My_Flags);
end;
```

would print:

`My_Flags are 111000100101;`

This section has shown that it is very straightforward to construct new `"and"` function for any user-defined data types, including aggregate types, and that once these new overloaded functions are visible they can be used in a formatting expression with the same conciseness and behaviour as the basic set of `"and"` functions.

4. Writing formatted text to other files

The features of the `Formatting_Text` package have, so far, been described in terms of delivering the result of the formatting onto Ada's `standard_Output` or `current_Output` files. This section describes the interfaces provided to deliver the formatted output into any other user-specified file. These interfaces allow the output to such files to be redirected or suppressed without changing or recompiling the uses of the interfaces.

Output of a formatted text string onto a user-specified file can be achieved by replacing the use of the `stdout` and `cout` functions with functions which have the same signature but which have been associated with a different file by instantiating the generic package shown in Table 10.

This generic package, which has no formal parameters, declares an object, named `Formatted`, of type `Formatted_File_Type`, derived from `Text_Io.File_Type,` to which the six functions, it also declares, are bound. Each function provides a different behaviour when the `Formatted` object to which they are bound is not open for writing. This behaviour is adopted throughout the evaluation of a single formatting expression which their invocation initiates.

The object `Formatted` is a visible object of a type derived from `Text_Io.File_Type` so that the user may apply any operations inherited from the `Text_Io` package to it; in particular, the file may be created, opened, closed and queried. The reasons for the object `Formatted` being declared in a generic package are discussed in section 7.2.

Table 10. The generic package to support output to any Text_Io.File_Type

```
generic
package Formatted_File is
   type Formatted_File_Type is new Text_Io.File_Type;
   Formatted    : Formatted_File_Type;
   Redirectable : Boolean := True;
   function File     (Format : string) return Formatter;
   function If_Open  (Format : string) return Formatter;
   function Redirect (Format : string) return Formatter;
   function File      return Formatter; -- uses the standard format "&s "
   function If_Open   return Formatter; -- uses the standard format "&s "
   function Redirect  return Formatter; -- uses the standard format "&s "
end Formatted_File;
```

4.1. The three types of Formatted_File functions

The purpose and behaviour of the three different functions are described below

4.1.1. The File function

The two forms of the **Formatted_File.File**, function provide exactly the same behaviour as the standard **Text_Io.Put** procedure in that if the **Formatted** object is not open the **exception Status_Error** will be raised. If the current mode of the file is not **Out_File** then the **exception Mode_Error** will be raised. Thus, formatting expressions initiated by this function will raise an exception if the **Formatted** object has not been previously opened for writing.

4.1.2. The If_Open functions

The functions **Formatted_File.If_Open**, on the other hand, will cause the result of the formatted expression, which they initiate, to be silently discarded when the associated **Formatted** object is not open with a **File_Mode** of **Out_File**. In fact, if the **Formatted** object is not open for writing when the **If_Open** function is executed then the formatting expression is not even evaluated; each operation called within the expression will immediately return without translating its arguments or interpreting its formatting string.

4.1.3. The Redirect functions

The functions **Formatted_File.Redirect** provide a halfway house between the two extremes provided above. If the **Formatted** object is not open for writing when the **Redirect** function is called then the result of evaluating the formatting expression, which it initiates, will depend upon the value of the Boolean **Formatted_File.Redirectable** as follows:

if **Formatted_File.Redirectable** = **False** then
    the result is discarded;

if **Formatted_File.Redirectable** = **True** then
    the result is redirected onto **Current_Output**; furthermore, the result will be redirected onto **Standard_Output** if **Current_Output** is closed.

4.2. Benefits of these functions

An advantage, that is provided by the above choices of behaviour for the output of text into a file, is that it becomes possible to associate different types of textual output with different instantiations of the generic **Formatted_File** package so that the actual generation, and output, of the text for these different files may be simply controlled by whether each file has been opened for writing at the time the corresponding formatted text statements are executed.

For instance, a system can be designed to have, say, four levels of diagnostic output. Each of these diagnostics levels can be represented by a separate instantiation of the **Formatted_File** generic package as shown in Table 11: The generation of diagnostic output at each of these four levels will then depend upon the status of their associated files; Table 12 shows what will happen if their files are not open when the diagnostic statements are executed.

Table 11. Using Formatted_File operations to control trace output

```
declare
   package   Level_1 is new Formatted_File;
   function Trace_1 (Format: string) return Formatter
                                 renames Level_1 .If_Open;
   package   Level_2 is new Formatted_File;
   function Trace_2 (Format: string) return Formatter
                                 renames Level_2.Redirect;
   package   Level_3 is new Formatted_File;
   function Trace_3 (Format: string) return Formatter
                                 renames Level_3.Redirect;
   package   Level_4 is new Formatted_File;
   function Trace_4 (Format: string) return Formatter
                                 renames Level_4.File;
begin
   Level_2.Redirectable := False;
   Put_Line (Trace_1 ("Entered My _Procedure"));
   Put_Line (Trace_2 ("Inputs are: &3{&s }") and x and y and z));
   Put_Line (Trace_3 ("Result is &s") and Answer);
   Put_Line (Trace_4 ("&s's entry (&s) count = &s")
                     and Entry_Name
                     and Entry_Index
                     and Entry'Count);
end:
```

Table 12. Effect of not opening output files

	Trace_1	Trace_2	Trace_3	Trace_4
File not open in package:	output:	output:	output	output
Level_1	suppressed			
Level_2 (Redirectable = False)		suppressed		
Level_3 (Redirectable = True)			Current Output	
Level_4				exception

5. Keeping the formatted text in memory

The facilities for formatting text have, so far, been described in terms of delivering the result directly to an Ada file. Whilst these facilities are likely to be sufficient for most applications they require that the text to be formatted is defined by a series of self-contained formatting expressions. Evaluating such formatting expressions may involve repeatedly re-evaluating some part of the expression which could be evaluated once and stored in memory for later use as part of several formatting expressions thereby saving both execution time and code space. For example, one may wish to associate with an error log some text that is particular to the source of the error but have a standard procedure that formats the bulk of the textual information; this is only feasible if one is able to retain formatted text strings in memory for later use in a formatting expression that is being delivered to an Ada file.

This section describes the interfaces that are provided, by the **Formatting_Text** package, to allow text strings to be formatted into records held in memory which may subsequently be used in other formatted text expressions.

To allow text strings to be stored in memory the **Formatting_Text** package defines the record type and operations shown in Table 13. An object of the record type **Text_Buffer_T** can store variable length Ada strings up to the maximum length defined by its discriminant **size**, which must have a fixed value specified for each object declared. The component **Current_Length** is used to define the index value of the last meaningful character position of the string currently held by the object in its **string_Part** component; it is set to zero when the object does not contain a meaningful **string_Part**. e.g. when such an object is declared.

5.1. Storing formatted strings in Text_Buffer_T objects

The four functions, shown in Table 13, are provided to allow the result of formatting expressions to be stored in **Text_Buffer_T** objects. These functions are used to initiate a formatting expression in exactly the same way as the file-based functions ; the functions **Into** write the formatted string into the specified **Text_Buffer_T** object whilst the functions **Append** append the formatted string onto the end of any **string_Part** the **Text_Buffer_T** already contains. If the **Text_Buffer_T** object is not big enough to hold the result of a formatting expression the **exception Text_Overflow** will be raised.

It should be noted that the **Text_Buffer_T** parameter has to be an **in** parameter, as it is a parameter of an Ada function, despite the fact that the value of this parameter is updated. This interface relies on parameters of a record type being passed by reference so that **T'Address** yields the address of the actual parameter, as defined in the LRM §13.7.2(15). Unfortunately, the Ada LRM §6.2:7 defines such an interface as erroneous. However, the author has yet to find an Ada compiler on which the above interface does not work and the use of a function, to specify the destination for a formatting expression, is essential to the integrity of the **limited private** type **Formatter**. For example, if the destination for a formatting expression was not known until after the expression had been evaluated the Formatting Buffer would need to be big enough to hold the whole formatted string and this is indeterminate. A number of alternative strategies were considered and discarded, as described in section 7.3.

Table 13. The interfaces for keeping formatted text in memory

```
type Text_Buffer_T (Size : Integer) is record
    Current_Length : Integer := 0;
    String_Part    : String (1 .. Size);
end record;

function Into   (T : Text_Buffer_T; Format : string) return Formatter;
function Append (T : Text_Buffer_T; Format : string) return Formatter;
function Into   (T : Text_Buffer_T) return Formatter; -- uses "&s "
function Append (T : Text_Buffer_T) return Formatter; -- uses "&s "
Text_Overflow : exception;

function "and"  (L : Formatter; R : Text_Buffer_T)    return Formatter;


procedure Put    (Into : in out Text_Buffer_T; From : String);
procedure Append (Into : in out Text_Buffer_T; From : String);
procedure Put    (Into :    out String;
                  From : Text_Buffer_T; Fill : Character := ' ');
```

5.2. New_Line operations

The only constraint that has been placed on storing formatted strings in memory is that the formatting control string must not specify any New_Line operations, i.e. it cannot contain any **&n** format control sequences. If one is encountered then the **exception New_Line_not_for_File** is raised. This constraint has been imposed to maintain portability of the package's behaviour.

Ada does not define how the New_Line operation is represented as an Ada string since different filing systems may need different character sequences. Consequently there is no standard representation for New_Line in Ada strings. The Formatting_Text package could have defined its own character string representation for New_Line operations stored in memory. This, however, would have meant that every string destined for a file would have had to have been scanned for this string representation so that they could be translated into the equivalent New_Line operations. This appeared to be an unacceptable run time overhead for very little extra functionality. In addition, defining an acceptable character string representation for New_Line operations would be fraught with difficulties.

5.3. Reading Text_Buffer_T objects in a formatting expression

To allow the **string_Part** component of a **Text_Buffer_T** object to be incorporated into a formatted string another overloading of the "**and**" operator is provided. This uses **R.String_Part (1 .. R.Current_Length)** as a string value in a formatting expression. Slices from **R.string_Part** can, of course, be referred to directly as string values in a formatting expression but they may then extract characters whose **string_Part** index exceeds the value in **Current_Length**.

The interfaces described above can be used to provide the facilities, described at the beginning of this section, whereby a general purpose Report_Error procedure, receives as a parameter, a formatted string it can use in a formatting expression. An example use of such an interface is given in Table 14; the function **Error_File** would, typically, be a renaming of an instantiation of the function **Formatted_File.Redirect**.

5.4 Other Text_Buffer_T operations

The other operations in Table 13. are provided to allow standard Ada string values to inter-operate with the **Text_Buffer_T** type. The procedure **Put** copies, and the procedure **Append** appends, their **From** string into the specified **Text_Buffer_T** object. If the **Text_Buffer_T** object is not big enough to hold the string the **exception Text_Overflow** is raised. The other **Put** procedure copies the **string_Part** from a **Text_Buffer_T** variable into the plain Ada string variable. If the **From.string_Part** is longer than the **Into** string it is truncated to fit; if it is shorter then the **Into** string is padded with the **Fill** character. This procedure can therefore never raise an exception.

Table 14. Example use of formatted text into memory

```
Put (Into (Text, "value &s of incorrect type") and Expected_Value);
Report_Error (Text, Line_No);
-- where:
procedure Report_Error (Text : Text_Buffer_T; Line_No : Integer) is
begin
-- can then contain:
Put_Line (Error_File ("Error on Line &d: &s") and Line_No and Text);
```

6. Formatting Calendar.Time

The formatting facilities, described in section 3, for user-defined data types could easily be applied to the Ada pre-defined type `calendar.Time` to construct an "and" function for such values that would deliver a standard textual representation of a `calendar.Time` value used in a formatting expression. This, however, would force all Calendar.Time values to have the same textual representation in all formatting expressions.

In ANSI C there are 21 conversion specifiers associated with time values that allow a wide range of textual representations of time to be composed from a format string by the function `strftime`. The need to provide flexibility in the textual formatting of time values has obviously been anticipated by these facilities in the C language; it was therefore thought to be advantageous to provide at least the equivalent flexibility over the textual representation of `calendar.Time` in Ada.

6.1. Translation of Date and Time values

To achieve this flexibility a formatting string has been defined for Date and Time values which uses the formatting notation that has already been described except that a different set of translation mode characters (conversion specifiers in ANSI C) are used. This formatting notation also supports all the layout features defined in Table 4. The translation mode characters that are applicable to Date and Time values are based on those defined by ANSI C and are shown in Tables 15 and 16.

The only ANSI C conversion specifiers not supported are c, C, x, X and Z since they can easily be composed from combinations of the other specifiers and Ada's Time does not support Time Zones. The translation mode characters D, f and s are not defined by ANSI C; D is a simple nicety of adding the ordinal suffix to the day of the month whilst f and s accommodate the fact that Ada's **Calendar.Time** has a resolution measured in fractions of a second and therefore allow seconds to be formatted as a real value.

Table 15. Translation Mode characters for Date values

Character	Interpretation	Formatting	Type	Example
a	Abbreviated weekday name	String		Wed
A	Full weekday name	String		Wednesday
b	Abbreviated month name	String		Mar
B	Full month name	String		March
d	Day of the month	range	1 .. 31	31
D	Day of the month with suffix	range	1 .. 31	31st
m	Month number	range	1 .. 12	3
j	day of the year	range	1 .. 366	62
U	Sunday week number	range	0 .. 53	10
w	weekday number (Sunday=0)	range	0 .. 6	3
W	Monday week number	range	0 .. 53	10
y	year number mod 100	range	0 .. 99	93
Y	year with century	range 1900 .. 2099		1993

Table 16. Translation Mode characters for Time values

Character	Interpretation	Formatting Type	Example
f	Seconds into Day (Duration)	range 0.0 .. 86400.0	34.567895
H	Hour of Day (24 hour Clock)	range 0 .. 23	22
I	Hour of Day (12 hour Clock)	range 0 ..12	9
M	Minutes into the hour	range 0 .. 59	45
p	a.m./p.m. indicator	String	am or pm
s	Full precision Seconds	range 0.0 .. 60.0	45.678875
S	Completed Seconds	range 0 .. 59	30

6.2. Date and Time formatting operations

These formatting facilities could have been provided as an Ada function with the specification: `function Date (Format : string; Time : Calendar.Time) return string`; which would be used in a formatting expression, thus:

```
Put_Line (Cout ("It is now &s")
      and Date ("&2_0H:&2_0M:&2_0S on &2_0d/&2_0m/&y", Calendar.Clock));
```

This may be regarded as adequate but suffers from the following problems:
- Every use of a `Calendar.Time` value in a formatting expression has to be accompanied by a Date formatting string and function call,

- Standard Date formatting strings would need to be defined in a package,
- Functions returning unconstrained strings are not necessarily efficiently implemented.

To overcome these shortcomings the generic package shown in Table 17 has been defined instead.

This generic package derives the type `Chronicle` from `calendar.Time` and defines a formatting "`and`" function for it. The package is instantiated with the formatting string that is to be applied to all instances of this derived type. The body of the function `Format_Chronicle` simply invokes a non-generic function that uses the `Chronicle_Format` with the `Chronicle` value to construct the required text into the `Formatting_Buffer` as needed by the instantiation of `And_User_Type`.

This approach allows the user to establish as many different Date and Time formats as are needed and ensures that the correct format is applied to the appropriate `Calendar.Time` derived type.

Table 17. Generic package specification for formatting Dates

```
function Format_Duration is new FT.And_Fixed (Duration);
generic
    Chronicle_Format : string;
package Chronometer is
    type Chronicle is new Calendar.Time;
    package FT renames Formatting_Text;
function Format_Chronicle (Into : FT.Formatting_Buffer;
                            This : Chronicle) return FT.Formatter;
function "and" is new FT.And_User_Type (Chronicle, Format_Chronicle);
function "and" (L : FT.Formatter; R : Duration) renames Format_Duration;
end Chronometer;
```

It also allows values of these types to be concisely used, like any other type, within a formatting expression, thus:

```
package Date is new Chronometer ("&2_0H:&2_0M:&2_0S on &2_0d/&2_0m/&y");
begin
    Put_Line (Cout and "It is now" and Date.Clock);
```

will produce:

```
    It is now 22:05:08 on 31/03/93;
```

The following two standard Date and Time formats are pre-instantiated:

```
package Full_Time is new   -- e.g. Wed, 31st March 1993 @ 22:05:08.200195
                        Chronometer ("&a, &D &B &Y @ &2_0H:&2_0M:&9_0s");

package Brief_Time is new -- e.g. 22:05:08 31 Mar 93
                        Chronometer ("&2_0H:&2_0M:&2_0S &d &b &2_0y");
```

6.3. A Timing interface

The above facilities for formatting `Calendar.Time` and `System.Duration` have been used to provide a Timing package with the following interfaces:

```
package Timers is
procedure Start (Log_Now : Boolean);
procedure Stop  (Log_Now : Boolean);
procedure Finish;
end Timers;
```

The package manages a stack of up to 50 concurrent timers, each of which is started by calling the procedure `Start` and stopped by calling the procedure `Stop`; the last Timer started is always the first Timer to be stopped. Elaboration of the package causes the statement:

```
Put_Line (Cout and Full_Time.Clock);
```

to be executed so that the program's output to `Cout` always contains a line recording the date and time of its execution.

If the `Boolean` parameter of the `Start` procedure is `True` the started Timer will immediately report, on `Current_Output`, the fact that a Timer has started with a message of the form:

```
Wed, 31st March 1993 @ 15:30:21.358024 started Timer N
```

This message will not be constructed, nor reported, if the `Boolean` parameter to the `Start` procedure is `False`.

If the `Boolean` parameter of the `Stop` procedure is `True` the Timer will be released for reuse after an elapsed time message has been sent to `Current_Output` of the form:

```
Wed, 31st March 1993 @ 15:30:33.123456 stopped Timer N after 11.765432 seconds
```

If, on the other hand, the `Boolean` parameter of the `Stop` procedure is `False` then no message is constructed and the Timer values are retained in memory and the Timer effectively remains in use until the `Finish` procedure is called. The `Finish` procedure sends to `Current_Output` the elapsed time message for all active and remembered Timers.

Setting the `Boolean` parameters to `False` allows up to 50 Timers to be used without the time taken to construct and output the timing reports distorting the figures that have been recorded. Setting the `Boolean` parameters to `True` allows up to 50 concurrent Timers and an unlimited number of sequential Timers to be used at the cost of the reported times and durations having to include the time taken to construct and output the messages. A reasonable estimate of the time taken to construct and output a pair of Timer start/stop messages can be obtained by starting two timers and immediately stopping them again.

7. Implementation considerations

This section discusses a number of alternative implementation policies that were considered during the development of the facilities described in this paper. The objectives for the implementation were to provide interfaces that were simply and concise to use, could be applied to any user defined type without loss of consistency and which generated minimal run time code when used. These objectives were sometimes in conflict with the features of Ada 83 which has led the author to adopt certain policies which may be frowned upon by Ada 83 purists. The following sections attempt to justify these policies as the only ones which satisfy these objectives and indicates where Ada 9X will provide features that support these policies.

Three aspects of the implementation are considered; the management of the buffers into which the text is temporarily formatted, using objects of Text_Io.File_Type as the destination for the formatted text and constructing the formatted text into memory.

7.1. Formatting Buffer management

Several policies for managing the Formatting Buffers which have to be used during the evaluation of a formatting expression were considered before the currently implemented policy was adopted. The various policies that were considered are discussed in this section to indicate why the current policy is considered, by the author, to be the best compromise for most application domains.

7.1.1. The problem to be solved

A Formatting Buffer is only active during the execution of either the `Put` or `Put_Line` procedure which take a parameter of type `Formatter`; values are not retained between statements. During the execution of these statements the Ada Run Time System may pre-emptively reschedule the Ada tasks causing another such statement to execute; the same statement could also be executed within the context of another Ada task. To cope with these possibilities it is necessary for the implementation of the formatting text facilities to be re-entrant, i.e.each invocation must have its own set of data objects. This means that a Formatting Buffer must not be shared by two or more formatting statements and must therefore be allocated at run time.

Ada data objects are allocated at run time by either:

* being declared as a local variable to a subprogram,
* the use of an allocator, i.e. being created on the heap.

This section discusses the characteristics of these two allocation policies and the policy that has implemented to achieve re-entrant management of the Formatting Buffers.

7.1.2. Stack-based buffers

The `Formatting_Text` package was prototyped with the use of buffers that had to be allocated by the user. It required each of the destination functions, such as `Sdtout`, `Cout`, `If_Open`, `Append` etc., to be given an additional `in out` parameter which identified the buffer to be used for the formatting expression evaluation.

This provided for re-entrant use of the facilities so long as the user did not use buffers declared at the package level; that is, the buffers had to be declared local to a subprogram. In practice, this meant that any subprogram that used the Formatting_Text facilities had to declare its own Formatting_Buffer object. This has a number of undesirable consequences which are discussed below:

7.1.2.1. Stack utilisation

The size of each subprogram's stack is increased by several hundred bytes (a Formatting Buffer typically requires about 250 bytes). These increased stack sizes can make a very significant contribution to the memory that has to be dedicated to the run time stack of each Ada task. During the execution of any task there will only ever be one Formatting Buffer object that is active since their use is restricted to be within a single formatting expression. All the space within the task's stack that has been allocated to other Formatting Buffers does not contain any useful values and is therefore space that is effectively never used. This can be unacceptable for Ada systems with limited memory resources.

7.1.2.2. Additional code

A Formatting Buffer contains records with discriminants. Therefore every Formatting Buffer object has to be initialised when it is elaborated. This code will form part of every subprogram that declares a Buffer and will be executed every time the subprogram is invoked unless the buffers are encapsulated in declare blocks with the formatting statements that use them.

Initialising the buffers could be avoided by using simpler data types within a Formatting Buffer at the cost of additional logic to manage the buffer.

7.1.2.3. Modification difficulties

Formatting Text statements are often used for diagnostic purposes and are therefore often only temporarily edited into a program. Such program source code editing is made more difficult and error-prone by the need to also edit the corresponding Formatting Buffer declarations. This editing could be simplified by the use of declare blocks but this would probably increase the number of buffer declarations and the subprogram's stack requirements.

It was therefore felt that the policy of requiring the user to declare the Formatting Buffers made the facilities less easy to use and introduced additional code and stack overheads.

7.1.3. Heap allocated buffers

The above shortcomings can be overcome by arranging for the implementation to allocate a Formatting Buffer on the heap at the start of a formatted expression evaluation and deallocating it on completion of the formatting statement. This simply requires that each destination function allocates a buffer and for the **Put** and **Put_Line** procedures to release it.

Now the user is not required to declare any buffers and memory is only allocated to a buffer when it is needed. In fact a program will only have more than one Formatting Buffer allocated simultaneously if a pre-emptive rescheduling occurs during the evaluation of one formatting expression and another starts executing concurrently. The memory space used to support the formatting of text is thereby minimised but at the cost of introducing the following undesirable consequences.

Performance overhead

With this policy each invocation of a text formatting statement involves the dynamic allocation, elaboration and deallocation of a Formatting Buffer. This is obviously an additional performance overhead on each execution of a text formatting statement.

Heap fragmentation

If a text formatting statement is executed without interruption then one would expect the management of the heap to be well-behaved in that no other heap operations will occur between the allocation and deallocation of the Formatting Buffer and the heap space should be immediately recovered and made available for other dynamic memory allocations.

If, on the other hand, the execution of a text formatting statement is interrupted the opportunity arises for other dynamic memory allocations to occur before the Formatting Buffer is released. Such interleaving of memory allocation and deallocation can lead to the fragmentation of the heap which requires the use of memory coalescing algorithms if a `Storage_Error` exception it to be avoided. The use of such algorithms make the behaviour of a program unpredictable which is unacceptable for embedded real time systems. It is for this reason that any repetitive dynamic allocation and deallocation of memory is best avoided for an embedded real time system.

It was therefore felt that the policy of allocating and deallocating Formatting Buffers on the heap every time a formatting expression is executed introduced the possibility of heap fragmentation and an unacceptable performance overhead.

7.1.4 Implementation management of the buffers

To minimise the performance and space overheads the implementation has adopted the policy of allocating a number of Formatting Buffers the first time that the facilities are invoked. The buffers are allocated the first time one is required rather than being allocated during elaboration of the package body so that the buffer space is not acquired when it is not needed, i.e. when a formatting expression is never evaluated.

The set of buffers is maintained in a circular list; each member of which indicates whether its buffer is currently is use or not. When a buffer is assigned to the evaluation of a formatting expression the "next available buffer" pointer is advanced round the circular list so that the next buffer is found as quickly as possible. It should be remembered that another buffer is only required if the evaluation of a formatting expression is interrupted by a pre-emptive rescheduling and another task starts executing a formatting expression.

This policy minimises the performance and space overheads at the cost of creating a small critical region of code that controls the state of these buffers. This critical region consists of the code which changes the status of a buffer when it is assigned to a formatting expression and there is a very small chance that this sequence of code is interrupted so that another thread of control could grab the same buffer:

```
if This.Target_Type = Not_in_Use then
    -- if interrupted here the same buffer may be assigned twice
    This.Target_Type := Not_Known;
```

The above problem can only be avoided, in Ada83, by the use of a task rendezvous and this was felt to be to heavyweight for these facilities. In Ada 9X protected records can be used to avoid this problem.

User control of Formatting Buffers

By default, the implementation allocates six Formatting Buffers the first time that a formatting expression is evaluated and if they all in use when another one is required the exception `No_Formatting_Buffers` is raised.

Facilities have been provided to allow the user to change this behaviour by controlling the number of buffers to be allocated, thus:

```
type Set_Buffers (Number:Integer; Unlimited:Boolean) is limited private;
```

The first discriminant, Number, is used to specify the number of buffers to be allocated when the first formatting expression is evaluated. The second discriminant, Unlimited, is used to specify whether further buffers are to be allocated as, and when, needed (Unlimited = True) or that no additional buffers are to be allocated Unlimited = False). Thus, the declaration:

```
The_Formatting_Buffers : Set_Buffers (Number => 3, Unlimited => True);
```

specifies that an initial allocation of 3 buffers is to be made and further buffers are to be allocated as, and when, needed. If this declaration is elaborated after a formatting expression has been executed then the default number of six buffers will already have been allocated.

The function:

```
function Buffers_Allocated return Integer;
```

is provided so that the user may establish the exact number of Formatting Buffers that have been allocated during the execution of a particular program when Unlimited has been set to true.

7.2. File_Type as a destination

To be able to write a formatted string into a `Text_Io.File_Type` as it is being constructed it becomes necessary to associate, in some way, the `File_Type` object with the `Formatting_Buffer` that is being passed through the formatted expression evaluation. The most natural way to achieve this would be to copy the value of a `File_Type` object into a component of the `Formatting_Buffer` object. This cannot be done since a `File_Type` is `limited private` and so a mechanism has to be found to overcome this constraint. This section describes several alternative approaches that were considered before the current use of a generic interface was implemented.

7.2.1. Access value to File_Type

Since values of a `File_Type` object cannot be copied one could resort to copying the value of an `access` type to a `File_Type`. This could be done with the following type of interface:

```
type Formatted_File is access Text_Io.File_Type;
function File     (File: Formatted_File;Format: string) return Formatter;
function If_Open (File: Formatted_File;Format: string) return Formatter;
function Redirect(File: Formatted_File;Format: string) return Formatter;
```

The value of the `File` parameter can now be copied into the `Formatting_Buffer` and passed through a formatting expression. However, the only way to associate the Boolean `Redirectable` with the `File_Type` object is now to construct a special record type to be used as the first parameter:

```
type Redirectable_File is
   The_File : Formatted_File;
   Redirectable : Boolean := False;
end record;
```

Now an object of this record type has be be declared by the user. If it is declared in the visible part of a package it is not sharable between tasks and cannot support re-entrant use of formatting expressions. If it is declared within a subprogram its visibility is limited and the `Redirectable` component cannot therefore be as easily controlled.

The other problem with using an `access` value is that is forces the user to allocate the `File_Type` objects on the heap which introduces the problems of memory management and garbage collection. These problems are usually not acceptable to long running programs with real time characteristics.

7.2.2. Reference to a File_Type

Another approach is to construct a reference to a File_Type object that is passed as an `in` parameter to the functions which have the following signatures:

```
function File     (File : File_Type; Format : string) return Formatter;
function If_Open  (File : File_Type; Format : string) return Formatter;
function Redirect (File : File_Type; Format : string) return Formatter;
```

However the interpretation of `File'Address` is undefined since it cannot be known whether the `limited private` type `Text_Io.File_Type` is a record type or an `access` type; in the latter case it is probable that `File'Address` will deliver the address of the parameter value rather than the address of the actual parameter. In addition, the only way to associate the Boolean `Redirectable` with the `File_Type` object is as described in section 7.2.1 which requires an `access` type to a `File_Type` to be constructed. Therefore this approach cannot avoid the use of an `access` value to a `File_Type`.

7.2.3. File_Type value as a package-level object

By forcing the `File_Type` object to be declared in the visible part of a package the Boolean `Redirectable` can be associated with it by simply declaring it as another visible object in the same package. The three functions `File`, `If_Open` and `Redirect`, which become visible operations of the package, are automatically associated with these two objects.

It now becomes possible for the implementation to rely on the operation `Formatted_File.Formatted'Address` always delivering the correct address which can be converted into `access` value referring to a `File_Type` object by use of an `Unchecked_Conversion`. This access value can be copied into the `Formatting_Buffer` and passed through the formatting expression as required. This approach will be able to be applied, without resorting to the use of `Unchecked_Conversion`, in Ada 9X by declaring the `Formatted_File_Type` to be an `aliased` subtype so that an `access` value to a statically allocated object may be obtained.

To ensure that this organisation is adhered to the package has been made `generic` with no formal parameters.

7.3. Text_Buffer_T as a destination

The interface described in section 5.2, for writing formatted strings into objects of the type `Text_Buffer_T`, relies on values of the type being passed by reference which, according to the Ada LRM, constitutes an erroneous program.

A number of alternative interfaces were considered to provide the facility to store a formatted string in `Text_Buffer_T` objects. These are described below with the reasons why they were rejected.

7.3.1. Generic object

An interface similar to that provided for `Text_Io.File_Type` could have been implemented as a generic package, thus:

```
generic
    Size : Integer;
package Formatted_Destination is
    type Formatted_Text is new Formatting_Text.Text_Buffer_T (Size);
    Buffer : Formatted_Text;
    function Into   (Format : string) return Formatter;
    function Append (Format : string) return Formatter;
    Text_Overflow : exception;
end Formatted_Destination;
```

This is safe as the `Into` and `Append` functions now implicitly write into the instantiated object `Formatted_Destination.Buffer`, but the user may need many instantiations and writing into `Formatted_Destination.Buffer` will not be sharable between tasks nor re-entrant.

7.3.2. Overloaded Put procedure

Since `New_Line` operations are not supported for `Text_Buffer_T` destinations, the procedure `Put_Line` will always raise an exception. Consequently only the procedure `Put` needs to be supported for `Text_Buffer_T` destinations and a special version could be implemented, thus:

```
Put (Destination : in out Text_Buffer_T, Formatted : Formatter);
function From (Format : string) return Formatter;
```

This interface would be used like this:

```
Put (Into(Text, From("value &s of incorrect type") and Expected_Value));
```

This, however, is not safe, since a `Formatter` value may already have been directed into a file, by use of the `cout` or `stdout` functions to construct a Formatter value. This insecurity could be overcome by introducing a new `limited private` type, thus:

```
type Format_Text is limited private;
Put (Destination : in out Text_Buffer_T, Formatted : Format_Text);
function From (Format : string) return Format_Text;
```

To provide the same functionality as for output to a `File`, one has to overload all the "`and`" functions and all the generics that instantiate "`and`" functions. This seems, to the author, a rather unnecessary replication of code to only achieve type-safety with no additional functionality.

7.3.3. Access values to Text_Buffer_T

The interface in section 5.2 treats the `in Text_Buffer_T` parameter to the `Into` and `Append` functions as a reference to a variable. The proper Ada mechanism to achieve this to use an `access` value as the parameter, thus:

```
type Text_Buffer_Ptr is access Text_Buffer_T;
function Into   (T : Text_Buffer_Ptr; Format : string) return Formatter;
function Append (T : Text_Buffer_Ptr; Format : string) return Formatter;
```

This, however, requires the users of the interface to use an allocator to create their `Text_Buffer_T` objects and therefore forces a program to use heap storage. This may not be appropriate for a long running embedded system with real time characteristics. Unless some form of garbage collection is employed `storage_Error`, due to lack of memory, will eventually occur. If garbage collection is employed then the real time responsiveness of a program will not be deterministic.

7.3.4. The implemented of a text formatting statement

Assuming that a parameter of a record type is passed by reference provides the simplest and most deterministic interface with the required type safety. Any other approach introduces unnecessary code and performance overheads at run time. Allowing Ada functions to have `in out` and `out` parameters would have allowed an appropriate interface to be legally implemented. In Ada 9X it will be possible to declare the `Text_Buffer_T` to be an `aliased` subtype so that an `access` value may designate a statically allocated object of the type.

8. Conclusions

The implementation policies that have been used have enabled the set of interfaces provided by the Formatting_Text package to be efficiently implemented in Ada 83. The package has been successfully compiled and used on several different Ada environments on different hardware architectures without having to change its source code. The package typically generates a target image of less than 15k bytes and each use of an overloaded `"and"` operator typically generates just a "push" and a "call" instruction.

The text formatting facilities provided by the package have been found to be very convenient, expressive and concise to use in practice with no loss of type safety. In this respect they are felt to be superior to the standard Ada Text_Io facilities and compare very favourably with the features of the standard Streams library of C++. The additional mechanisms available in Ada 9X will allow these formatting facilities to be "correctly" implemented and , it is to be hoped, without loss of efficiency.

The author wishes to acknowledge his indebtedness to Steve Sutton (now at CSA Systems Ltd, Auckland N.Z.) for his contribution to , and his constructive evaluation of, the many experimental prototypes that preceded the current interfaces and implementation. His conviction that "it should be easier to use than this" was a constant stimulus to the development of this package.

Sudden Infant Death Syndrome monitoring on a lap-top using Ada

Chris HALL

Department of Applied Computing and Electronics
Bournemouth University, Talbot Campus, Poole, BH12 5BB, Dorset. UK.

Abstract. This paper describes a system developed to support the work of an academic paediatrics research unit conducting a large scale clinical study of Sudden Infant Death Syndrome. The system provides for the acquisition, archiving, analysis and viewing of physiological data. An Apple lap-top with a low-cost slaved interface unit is responsible for acquiring the data at the cot-side during over-night studies. The acquired data is then processed and analysed on a large screen Apple computer system. The clinicians are provided with processing and graphical tools which will allow them to move quickly through the mass of data to identify periods of interest relevant to their studies. All the software for the project has been developed in Ada. The paper discusses the benefits of using Ada for such a project and also describes the experience of using the language on a general purpose lap-top computer.

1. Introduction

Sudden Infant Death Syndrome (SIDS) is a phenomenon which has caused deep distress in society for countless years. Many research groups are currently searching for the contributory cause(s). One of the important aspects of any study of this kind is to base any conclusions on as wide a study sample as possible. For this reason the clinical study associated with this project requires overnight monitoring of the majority of infants passing through the maternity unit of a major hospital during a period of years. Each overnight study may last up to 12 hours with thousands of babies being monitored during the period of the full study.

An overnight study will typically monitor physiological parameters such as ECG, pulse, respiration, airflow, transcutaneous skin-oxygen levels and blood oxygen saturation. The sampling rates, selection of channels and signal conditioning, however requires flexibility and the facility for easy change as the study progresses. The large number of studies require analysis and comment by the clinicians and subsequent archiving for future reference. The clinicians require a way of navigating through the mass of data to identify periods of interest which may last for less than 2 minutes in a 12 hour study. In earlier studies of shorter periods, recordings have been output on analogue chart recorders and clinician have to flipped through the charts in their search for relevant sections. This can take tens of minutes even with short recordings. In the full scale project this time is not available.

The software developed provides clinicians with a 'big picture' of the complete recording period allowing them to home in on important events very quickly. Their comments can then be entered on-line and archived with the full recording on optical disk.

As the project develops it is planned to provide automatic analysis of the recordings and further speed up the task of the clinician.

2. The computers and the choice of Ada

The choice of Apple [1] computers was prompted by the experience of these machines by the paediatrics team. The well proven and established graphical user interface (GUI) of the Macintosh supported by the very capable systems architecture of the Macintosh operating environment made it an ideal and flexible platform on which to base the software.

The choice of development language was unconstrained. Conventional or popular wisdom might have pointed to 'C' as the obvious choice. Perversely Ada was selected:

- as a case of 'doing as I preach' - why should the teacher use different methods to those advocated to undergraduates;

- to evaluate the use of ada as a development vehicle for low-end general purpose computers, possibly repudiating the apocryphal stories of slow run-time, and enormous run-time systems and generated code;

- to investigate how successfully Ada software could integrate with and use the low-level facilities of an interactive event-driven system;

- to exploit the provision for multi-tasking; and

- to prove a personal conviction that Ada provided a better chance of delivering the software on-time even on low-end personal computers - an experience not enjoyed by the author with previous projects using C.

3. Description of system

A schematic diagram of the total system is shown below.

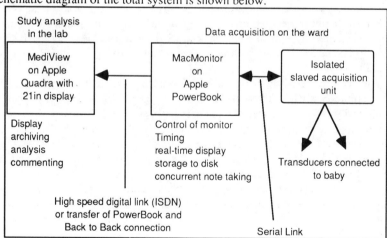

Fig. 1 Schematic of baby monitoring System

The system consists of two main units: the first consisting of an Apple PowerBook running the MacMonitor software and communicating with a purpose built module containing all the electronics for signal conditioning, digital to analogue conversion and satisfying all the stringent conditions for electrical isolation; the second is the main signal viewing workstations used by the medics for examining the overnight recordings. This is a standard Apple Quadra running the MediView software.

3.1. Data acquisition and MacMonitor

A major influence on the design of the system was the need to keep the slaved acquisition unit simple, minimising specialist hardware and retaining all timing functions and the selection of sampling rates and channel selection totally within the lap-top software. The lap-top communicates with the slave unit over an optically isolated but otherwise standard serial link. The acquisition box contains a simple Mitsubishi microcontroller and behaves in a totally subordinate role. The total reliance on the lap-top for sample timing and channel selection made it essential that the lap-top software could guarantee accurate timing with no incremental creep over an extended period, in parallel with the other functions it was required to provide.

The MacMonitor software performs the following functions:
* Initial input of baby's details from nurse or doctor
* initialisation of slaved acquisition unit
* selection of sampling characteristics and channel selection based on acquisition unit type (derived from initial dialogue) and study required
* *continuous and accurately timed requests to the acquisition unit for samples*
* *archiving of data blocks to hard disk*
* *real-time display of physiological traces on screen*
* *operator entry of event notes concurrent with above.*
* study termination determined by the nurse/doctor.

The functions detailed in italics need to be handled concurrently with the guarantee of accurate control of the sampling being critical. In practice this relies on sampling request codes being fired at the acquisition unit controlled by a central timing task. All other software functions are considered subordinate to this. Each channel may be sampled at a different rate dependent on the study and the nature of the physiological channel being monitored.

The acquired data (c 6Mbytes for a 12 hour recording) is then compressed (typically 4:1) and then transferred to the viewing workstation. The transfer is accomplished either by modem or ISDN connection, or if the monitoring session was conducted on the same site, by physically taking the PowerBook and connecting it back to back as a SCSI device to the main workstation.

3.2. Study viewing and MediView

The MediView software is designed to allow the clinician to navigate through a large quantity of physiological data for events of interest. The software enables the user to view and compare several studies or different views of the same study simultaneously, each in a separate window. The user can select appropriate time scales, combination of traces to display, and the type of automatic feature recognition to be used.

The software conforms to the Apple GUI guidelines and provides a multiple windows environment with a window attached to each monitoring session the clinician is studying. Because of the large quantity of data being handled and the lengthy processing times (relative to patience of a typical clinician) each window is supported by Ada tasks enabling the processing of data to be handled concurrently with other more interactive tasks.

Normally when a clinician calls for display of processed information this will have been completed whilst they were studying other displays, minimising the user wait times.

Both MediView and MacMonitor make significant use of the Macintosh resource based nature of application construction to allow close integration of the two items. When MacMonitor archives data to disk files it also includes resource objects which contain information on sampling rates and channels selected in addition to the baby's details. This resource object being passed with the data enables the software to be far more flexible, allowing single versions of both to cope with varied requirements and also enable changes to be made relatively painlessly by medical technicians.

4.   General principles of the software design

The central principles behind the software design were:
*   to fully exploit the benefits of the Ada language such as strong typing, tasking, generics, overloading etc.;
*   to keep within the security of the Ada language environment and restrict to an absolute minimum excursions to assembler, or C;
*   to adhere to the Apple GUI guidelines; and
*   to make full use of the built-in Apple operating environment facilities such as the separation of logical objects through the use of resources.

5.   Overview of the Macintosh platform

To some extent the first two general design principles of staying within the Ada environment are in conflict with the third and fourth principle of fully exploiting the Apple environment. This requires a carefully thought out way of interfacing the two 'worlds' not simply in terms of the code interfaces but also the dynamic structure of the software - not least the problem of interfacing the world of GUI and other events to the Ada world of tasks and the rendezvous.

The next section will discuss these issues in more detail, however, it is useful here to present a summary of the main features of the Apple environment.
*   The Apple operating system provides an effective cooperative multi-processing environment with full support for inter-process communication.
*   The main interface between the OS and the application software is through events and event queues. These events may be derived from hardware, window activities and application generated communications.
*   The 'standard' look and feel of apple software is derived from the adherence to GUI standards and the use of the 'Tool-box' facilities provided in the OS. All software developers are encouraged to work through this tool-box.
*   In the Apple domain all software is seen as a collection of resources. From the early days of the original Macintosh the system has encouraged the logical separation of objects such as windows, window drawing functions, strings, palette definitions, etc., from the control code which manipulates the objects. This approach leads to easy localisation of software and in the case of the MediView and MacMonitor applications, maintenance of key areas of the software by non-computer skilled users.
*   Key interrupt triggered functions such as time-up or disk transfer finished are handled by 'call-back' routines, traditionally written in assembler or Pascal.

6.   Fusing the Ada and Apple worlds

This section focuses on the three major issues tackled in the monitoring software: interfacing the OS and GUI world of events and interrupts to the Ada tasking model within MediView; relating to and utilising the object based resource features of the Macintosh environment; and finally the problem of ensuring concurrency and timeliness with an application running on an ordinary lap-top computer.

6.1   Interfacing OS events to the Ada tasking model

Fig. 2. shows a typical viewing screen where the paediatrician is analysing a mixture of monitoring sessions, showing different trace combinations, periods, timebases and subjects.

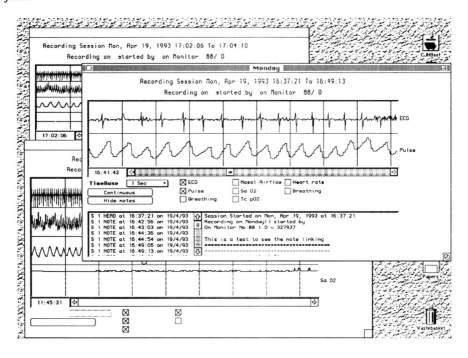

Fig. 2. Screen capture showing multiple session windows in use

Each monitored session being viewed is seen as logically independent and autonomous and each session related window is 'looked after' by a separate task (Fig. 3). One of the problems with working with large quantities of data is that it can take some time to process the data (for example to derive heart rate from the ECG) prior to display. In order to deliver a crisp response the system tries to anticipate the periods of a session the viewer will move to next. To enable this processing each session task spawns a child task trying to make sure that processed data is already available when it is requested. These children operate at low priority as background tasks, with the tasks relating to the front or active window receiving precedence.

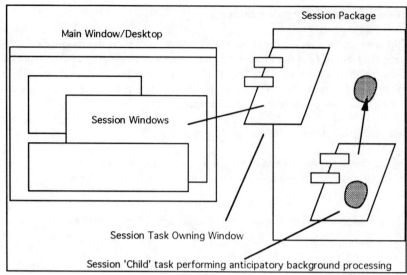

Fig. 3. Session Tasking Structure

When looking at the dynamics of the session task it is clear that most of the messages it receives will derive from the external world relating normally to user activated requests. The screen dumps in Fig. 2 show that the windows contain many user controls such as buttons, scroll bars, selection boxes and lists. All of the user requests need to be translated into rendezvous messages directed at the appropriate session task entry point.

To appreciate the operation of this interface requires some description of the Apple operating system and event handling (Fig 4.) Although events may originate from many different sources the application receives them via a single event queue maintained by the Operating System. There is an event queue for each running application and it is the responsibility of the application to ensure that this queue is interrogated frequently enough to give satisfactory user response. This would normally mean checking to see if any events are waiting about 60 times per second.

Although the operating system's toolbox event manager maintains these queues the actual events are derived from a variety of sources. Most of them will ultimately have originated as interrupts, however, software managers handle these and convert them to event messages.

A summary of the events and their use is as follows -

- High level events are intended for inter-application communication including networked distributed applications. MediView receives them only from the 'Finder' (OS shell) when a user opens a data file (double-clicks a file icon). In this case the accompanying event message details the file identity.
- Process manager derived. The Apple system uses cooperative multi-tasking and if the user selected an alternative application the Finder would send Suspend events to the active application. The awakening application receives a resume event.
- Window events. If an alternative window is selected the window manager sends the appropriate pair of window de-activate and window activate messages to the appropriate application. It also keeps track on visible window drawing regions and if these change a window update event may be sent.

- Key and Mouse events are first placed into a common event queue which the Toolbox event manager unpacks into the application specific queues.

Although the baby monitoring applications makes use of and handles nearly all possible event types the most frequent are window or mouse related.

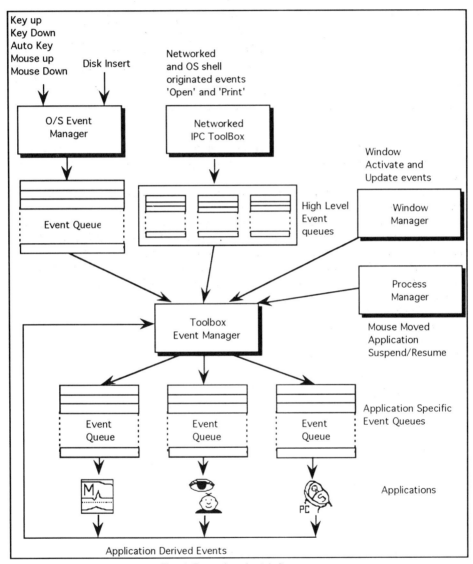

Fig. 4. Events into the Ada Programs

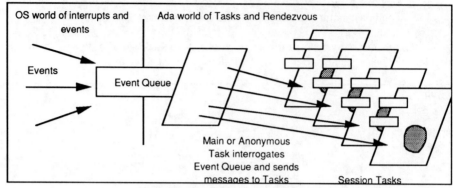

Fig. 5. Directing OS events to session tasks

This event handling structure presents two problems: one of relating an event to the task responsible and secondly scheduling to ensure that all activities receive the time they need.

When the user requests to open a session file the anonymous main task dynamically creates a session record and session task. This is then sent an open message which causes the task to open the file, initialise the corresponding data structures and create a window. All system window control blocks, as do most system control blocks, contain a user defined data area. This has a copy of the session task access object placed into it. When a window related event is retrieved from the queue by the main task it uses this control block entry to identify the owning session task to which to send the message (Fig. 5 schematic, Fig.6 code framework).

```
PROCEDURE MediView is

      PROCEDURE DoEvent(event: Events.EventRecord) IS
         BEGIN
            CASE event.what IS
               -- selects those events which are processed in anonymous task e.g New_task,close and
quit
               -- and actions them
               --else it identifies owning session task and sends it a message
            END CASE;
         END DoEvent;

      PROCEDURE EventLoop IS
         BEGIN
            LOOP  -- forever, or at least Quit
               gotEvent    :=       Events.WaitNextEvent(       -- obtain next event
                     mask      =>      Events.SelectEventMask,  -- selects events of interest
                     event     =>      Event,                   -- returned event message
                     sleep     =>      0,                       -- don't wait if no event
                     mouseRgn  =>      NULL);                   -- ignore
               IF gotEvent THEN DoEvent(event); END IF;

               DELAY 0.017;        -- Give way to enable other tasks time to run and at least 1/60th
Sec

               SystemTasks;        -- Give way to OS to enable periodic OS functions to execute

            END LOOP;
         END EventLoop;

BEGIN
   Initialize;                -- initialize program
   Display_About_Dialog;      -- application launch screen
   EventLoop;                 -- enter main event loop
END MediView;
```

Fig. 6. Eventloop framework in main anonymous task

```
PACKAGE Session IS

    TASK TYPE Session_Task_t  IS
        -- Entry specifications
        ENTRY start(myTask_rec_AC_p  :   IN     Task_rec_AC_t;
                    FileSpec          :   IN     FSSpecPtr;
                    Result            :   OUT    Task_Error_t) DO

    END Session_Task_t;

    TYPE Session_rec_t IS  Session record specification
        RECORD
            Task  :  Session_Task_t; -- Session owning task
            -- window and session related objects

        END RECORD;

    -- subprogram specifications
    PROCEDURE  DoOpen(FileSpec  : IN    FSSpecPtr);  -- creates new session record and task
                                                     -- and opens data window opens file

END Session;
PACKAGE BODY Session IS

    PROCEDURE  DoOpen(FileSpec  :  IN    FSSpecPtr)  IS
        -- creates new task and opens data window opens file
        BEGIN
            -- dynamic creation of session record and new task (New_Task function)
            Current_Task_AC  := New_Task;
            IF Current_Task_AC /= NULL
                THEN
                    Current_Task_AC.Task.Start(myTask_rec_AC_p    =>   Current_Task_AC,
                                               FileSpec           =>   FileSpec,
                                               Result             =>   Error);
                    -- Send start message and pass over session file details
                    IF Error /= NoErr THEN --Error handling routines END IF;
            END IF;
        END DoOpen;

    TASK BODY Session_Task_t IS
        -- Task local objects and local type declarations and Task local subprograms

    BEGIN
        SELECT
            -- task must initially wait for start message with file details
            ACCEPT start  (myTask_rec_AC_p  :   IN     Task_rec_AC_t;
                           FileSpec          :   IN     FSSpecPtr;
                           Result            :   OUT    Task_Error_t) DO
        END SELECT;

        --  Now enter main loop of task
        WHILE Task not flagged as dying LOOP
            SELECT
                ACCEPT Mouse_Event(  event :   IN     Events.EventRecord;
                                     part  :   IN     short_integer) DO
                    -- adjust stack to save area
                    Old_Stack    := Capture_SP;
                    Set_SP(Stack_Base);     -- adjust stack to save area
                    -- invoke apropriate routines
                    Set_SP(Old_Stack);      -- restore stack
                END Mouse_Event;
            OR
                -- Other message accept points
            END SELECT;
            DELAY 0.0;  -- give way to other tasks
            -- service child processing task if necessary
        END LOOP;
END Session;
```

Fig. 7. Framework of session task

The Apple system is designed for single user workstations and does not implement time-sliced preemptive scheduling. It provides a cooperative multi-tasking process manager which places the onus on the running applications to 'give way' in a responsible manner. The Ada run time system does, however, provide the choice of either pre-emptive or non-preemptive scheduling of Ada tasks. At the MediView design stage there was therefore a clear tension in which scheduling method to select, as summarised below.

- The MediView application has to ensure that it interrogates the event queue sufficiently regularly to give adequate response time.
- MediView must periodically (at least once per second) give way to allow system functions or other background applications a chance to run.
- It must give all session tasks adequate time to maintain the displayed data.
- The child of each session task must be given some background time to process data.

It was tempting to use the preemptive scheduling of the Ada run time system to ensure a 'fair' distribution of time, however, it was considered safer and more efficient to take on the responsibility for scheduling within the application and opt for non-preemptive. Another more pragmatic reason was that the tasking mechanism and the placement of task stacks creates problems for Apple graphics toolbox (QuickDraw), requiring a small fix described in a later section. This made it more important to opt for a totally determinate method. The Figs. 6 and 7 program outlines indicate where these give way points occur.

6.1   Relating to the Object based resource structure of the Macintosh

The project was originally started with a specific study in mind, however, it was clear at the outset that this type of medical monitoring system has got many and varied potential applications. If this potential was to be realised it was clear that future applications should be encompassed with no or minimal change to the basic programs but should be achieved by tailoring by medical technician staff with no knowledge of the esoteric world of Ada. As will be seen from the conclusions this objective has been satisfied.

To achieve this objective required an object oriented design philosophy to be adopted of logically separating the control structures and operations from the objects on which they operate and to enable these objects to be manipulated post system development by technicians. Essentially this means not embedding within the code of the program any definitions or structures on which it will operate. The object oriented debate is clearly very topical at the current time, however, much of the OO nature and ease of modification in this system is achieved through exploiting the object oriented nature of the Macintosh System architecture.

Arising out of the early work at Palo Alto the Macintosh from the outset encouraged the logical separation of objects from the control structures. In the Macintosh environment these objects and the associated methods are called resources.

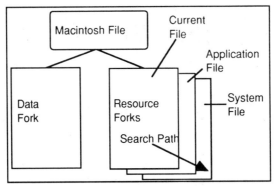

Fig. 8. Macintosh resource system

Any Macintosh file (Fig 8) has two parts known as the data and resource forks. For a typical data file the resource fork is empty whilst for a typical application file the data fork is empty. Resources are basically the data objects such as windows, strings of text, images, graphical control buttons which an application manipulates and the 'methods' or code procedures which operate on them. When a resource (either an object or a method) is specified by the running application the operating system searches the current file's resource fork first, if one is not found there it then searches the applications own resource fork and finally it resorts to the system's own resource fork. This order establishes an important principle that if an alternative resource is not provided by the user or application the system default will be used. An example - the application creates a new window, the windows size, colour shape will be specified in a the resource fork of the application. The code or 'method' governing the way the window will be drawn is left to the system's own default method in the system's resource fork. If out of perversity we wanted an unusual behaviour for a window we could develop our own methods and add this as a resource in the application or data file resource fork. This would then override the system's default.

Resources can either be variations of existing system defined resources or user defined. In the case of MacMonitor and MediView two additional sets are created over and above the standard. The first contains a specification of sampling rates, channel names, display characteristics, scaling factors etc. for each of the variations of monitoring studies. As new variations are introduced the only change required is the addition of new versions of this basic resource. A great benefit of this technique is that these resources may be created with very limited computer knowledge. A utility program called a resource editor (ResEdit[2]) can be used against a template to allow technicians to create a new version or modify an existing one. Fig 9. shows the collection of resources contained in MediView. The appearance of the user interface, the sounds used, the control of sampling rates can all be determined or changed by using ResEdit. Little knowledge of the program is necessary, purely the skill to drive the graphically based editor of the tool.

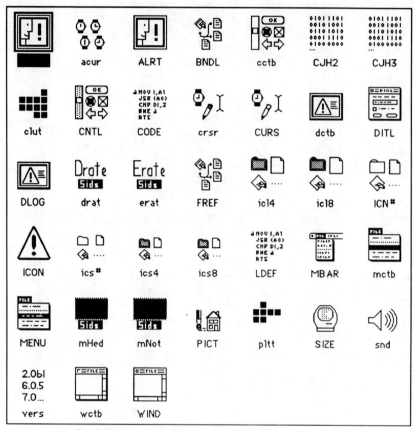

Fig. 9. MediView seen by ResEdit as a collection of Resources

Fig 10 shows the template view which a medical technician would see when modifying or constructing a new monitoring regime.

The same application defined resource technique is used for the addition of session information and notes added dynamically during a recording. These are added to the data file as 'note' resources and form a linked list. They become an integral part of the file and MediView allows the user to step through these notes moving to points of interest in the recording.

Manipulating resources from Ada presents little problem. The OS resource manger toolbox provides subprograms to access the resources. All of the system defined resources have record mappings included with the Ada interface library. In the case of the user defined resources mapping records had to be created for use within the Ada programs, and also template specification resources prepared using ResEdit and incorporated into ResEdit resource fork to enable subsequent users to access these resources in the form shown in Fig. 10.

```
Master          64
Sampling
rate

No of           8
Channels

1) *****

Channel Name    ECG

Channel rate    1

Initial         1
Display mode

Colour of       20
trace (CLUT
pos)

Maximum         10
valid
timescale

Scale Factor    1

Minor           0
graduations

Major           0
graduations

When 0          0
sampled
channel
or Res no of
processing
code

If derived -    0
Related
```

Fig. 10. ResEdit template view enabling modification or creation of new sampling control resource

6.1 Concurrency and timeliness on a Lap-top

MacMonitor the lap-top software has four activities which it must handle concurrently. These are listed below in order of their time critical nature.

1. Sending sampling requests to the baby interface unit. The mix of samples requested varies, however, the timing and the regularity must be consistent and in line with the specification found in the sampling resource 'erat'.

2. Data must be written to screen to provide the nurse/doctor with a continuous display of life functions. The display must be smooth with no jerks.

3. Data must be archived periodically to hard disk without affecting 1) and having little effect on 2).

4. On demand the user can request a dialogue entry box to record an event note indicating such things as the administering of medication or some physiological observation. This interaction with the user must not interfere with either 1 or 3.

On analysis, only activity 1 is very time critical in the sense that any delay or time inaccuracy would invalidate the data sampling process. The other activities can suffer short scheduling delays causing few problems other than an occasional jerk in the screen display or a short delay in responding to a user's key press when entering a note.

The time critical activity 1 is effectively interrupt driven, however, the Ada code is kept well away from this level. The normal method of linking a task entry point to a timer interrupt could not be used as this capability is not implemented in the Ada system used. The OS does, however, provides a time manager. This is issued with time delay requests which are queued in time expiry order. The expiry time can be linked to a 'call-back' routine, which can hence be programmed to perform the time dependent activity. The time manager, although not guaranteeing accurate call-back to the µSec, does modify the time interval to take any slight drift into account thus ensuring no long term creep. The call-back routine is written totally in Ada, the only need being a short generic glue routine written in C to tie the Pascal based OS world to the Ada routine. The call-back routine sends out the appropriate request to the slaved interface unit, then places a copy of the request into a circular buffer so that it can be tied up with the returning samples by the normal event loop activities of the main program.

The other three activities are handled in the normal event loop model. This loop is exercised at least 60 times a second. Observing the precedence of the activities, it checks the incoming data stream from the baby interface, checks them for integrity against the samples requested, then both outputs to the screen and file buffer. When the file buffer is full an asynchronous write request is queued to the OS so that archiving can then proceed in parallel with the other continuing tasks. When the user requests an entry note, MacMonitor makes visible a latent entry dialogue box on the screen and allows future key down events to be passed to the dialogue manager until the note is complete. Other activities continue throughout this period.

7.   Performance of the system and critical evaluation of software

7.1   Development environment

The software has been developed using an Apple Quadra 700 (25Mhz 68040 with 12Mbyte memory and 160Mbyte disk) and also a Apple IIci (25MHz 68030 with 20Mbyte and 230Mbyte disk). The Ada environment used is Meridian Ada version 4.1.5 from Meridian Software Systems. This runs on top of the Macintosh Programmers Workbench (MPW) version 3.2. This is multi-window development environment which also supports 'C', C++ Pascal and assembler.

The Macintosh Meridian Ada comes complete with a full set of interface packages which conform closely with those specified by the 'Inside Macintosh'[3] technical reference series published by Apple. A minor problem arose when the interface library supplied with version 4.1 did not cover the extra and important features included in Apple's new version of the operating system - version 7. This presented few problems as it proved to be very straightforward to build the Pragma interface packages to use these features prior to the release of version 4.1.5 which corrected the deficiency.

In some situations an instrumentation package LabVIEW 2.1.5 from National Instruments was used to prototype[4] and test algorithms and also to simulate the baby interface unit in the absence of hardware. This package which uses a visual programming paradigm enabled this work to proceed more quickly prior to their final inclusion in the Ada programs.

7.2   System statistics

There are many horror stories of the size and slow speed of programs developed in Ada. These have certainly not been shown in this project. MediView is currently c10,000 lines of code and MacMonitor about 5,000. This does not take into account the definition of the non-code resources the programs use.

Program	Executable Size	Code Resource Size	No of Code resource Modules	User defined Resource	Opening Dialogue Screen	Running Requirements
MediView	271,302b	124,456b	51	c30,000b	88,538b	>3Mb
MacMonitor	65,284b	33,254b	30	c17,000b	8,000b	c500kB

Table 1. Program statistics.

Table 1 shows that both the executable program and the code   sizes are very reasonable and in the authors experience don't greatly exceed those expected with the equivalent programs developed in 'C' or Pascal. It is also significant that with the growing trend for colourful and eye catching start up screens, these significantly increase the file size (MediView has captured images of babies and these occupy >88,000 bytes or over 25% of the executable file size).

User defined resources have been specified either textually using a resource compiler which comes with MPW or by using ResEdit with which they can be built graphically. The sound resources used for audible warning of events were captured using the inbuilt sound facilities of the Macintosh system.

Although much of the software works very closely with the operating system and the physical machine, with interrupt time call-back routines and off-screen drawing being used, out of the total 15,000 lines of code it has only been found necessary to desert Ada on extremely rare occasions. There are a few (<5) small 'C' written glue routines to tie in call-back routines and there are also two functions used to overcome task stack problems where two machine code instructions are used. The vast majority of the software delivers the required performance with the full run-time error checking and exception mechanisms active. Only in a small area of the information processing intensive parts of the program has the Pragma suppress been used to gain some 50% speed improvement.

Out of interest the interface to the OS functions from the Ada environment has also be scrutinised. The Ada parameter passing mechanisms are very similar to the Pascal type mechanisms used in the Apple OS. The linkage through the hardware Trap mechanism is hence extremely efficient.

7.3   Specific Problems

The Macintosh system environment although very powerful and complete is inherently complex hence it is not straightforward to develop software to sit on this platform. The majority of the problems encountered were not generally produced by the use of Ada but by coming to terms with the Macintosh environment. Once these were well understood the design of the Meridian Ada Interface packages make it relatively straightforward to build software. There were however several specific problems which are worthy of note.

Firstly Meridian Ada, quite reasonably, when creating tasks dynamically using task access types, reserves unique storage space for the task to use as its stack, and this area is taken from the general program heap storage. The vast majority of the time this causes no problem, however, an undocumented 'feature' of QuickDraw the Apple graphics manager is that it checks the position of the stack when it receives some (not all) graphics drawing requests and if it does not conform to its idea of where the stack should be it does nothing. It does not make the program fall over or generate error reports it simply leads to windows being drawn in a bizarre way. This problem/feature was overcome by the task switching its stack to a safe area prior to any system function involving graphics (Fig 5). This fix has proven to be very effective and reliable, however, it does raise questions about the use of preemptive scheduling with tasks using graphics.

Secondly the MacMonitor program was developed to run on a PowerBook 100, the first of the Apple Lap-tops. This only has a passive matrix LCD display and also a relatively slow processor clock speed of about 10MHz. MacMonitor performs perfectly happily within these constraints until the user requests input of a dynamic note when it ran out of time to maintain all the concurrent tasks. The simply remedy of detecting the machine type running the program has been adopted. If it is a PowerBook 100 it suspends the data display activity. On the more recent and more powerful machines this does not present any problem.

8.   Conclusions

The software is now in use with the original sudden infant death syndrome study in the Department of Academic Paediatrics at Stoke City General Hospital.

As predicted the need for such a system is proving to be quite wide spread. The generic design [5][6] has enabled several other variations of the basic system to be introduced for separate studies within the original research group. For example one system is being introduced to monitor cerebral blood flows using near infrared spectroscopy, and another is being used in an ambulatory monitoring project observing EEG traces in infants with suspected fits. Versions are also being introduced into other projects in Jamaica in the W. Indies and Hanover in Germany.

The ease with which these studies have been accommodated demonstrates the success of the original design strategy. Very little change has been necessary to the original design of the software, the majority being accomplished through modifying or adding new resources.

This project demonstrates that Ada is not just a vehicle for large-scale multi-man system development but has very significant advantages in small scale projects based on low-cost personal computers. Although controlled comparisons could not be made, the size of the software produced and its run-time performance were little different to what might be expected in similar applications developed in other languages. The benefits of using Ada, however, in terms of ease of implementation, enabling a better and more logical abstraction of the problem domain, and minimising debugging time were very significant.

The author believes that because of the use of Ada the software produced is of higher quality. It has certainly proved possible to deliver the required performance on time with few bugs being reported by the clinicians using the system. This judgement is subjective, however, and will remain so until the software has been in use over a longer period when maintenance figures may be used as more tangeable metric.

The project demonstrates that it is possible to build applications on standard low-cost microcomputer environments without undue compromise exploiting the strengths of both the Ada language and the power and facilities of the underlying system architecture.

9. References

[1] Apple Computer Inc. Technical Introduction to the Macintosh Family. Addison Wesley, 1987

[2] Alley,.P & Strange, C. ResEdit Complete. Addison Wesley 1991

[3] Apple Computer Inc. Inside Macintosh family. Addison Wesley.

[4] Hall, C.J. & Burns. R System development and integration without pain using LabVIEW on the Macintosh Apple HE 93 Conference. St Andrews.

[5] Hall, C.J. & Holder, A.S. Generic system for the acquisition, archiving and analysis of physiological data Biomed 93 Conference. Bath. UK

[6] Hall, C.J. & Holder, A.S. Low-cost system for the acquisition, archiving and visualisation of physiological data in large scale clinical projects. Health Care Computing 93. Harrogate, UK